Astrology

FOR

Wellness

Astrology

FOR

Wellness

Star Sign Guides for Mind, Body & Spirit Vitality

MONTE FARBER & AMY ZERNER

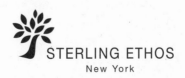

STERLING ETHOS
New York

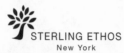

STERLING ETHOS
New York

An Imprint of Sterling Publishing Co., Inc.
1166 Avenue of the Americas
New York, NY 10036

STERLING ETHOS and the distinctive Sterling Ethos logo are
registered trademarks of Sterling Publishing Co., Inc.

Text © 2019 The Enchanted World of Amy Zerner & Monte Farber
Cover © 2019 Sterling Publishing Co., Inc.

ISBN 978-1-4549-3246-8

Distributed in Canada by Sterling Publishing Co., Inc.
c/o Canadian Manda Group, 664 Annette Street
Toronto, Ontario M6S 2C8, Canada
Distributed in the United Kingdom by GMC Distribution Services
Castle Place, 166 High Street, Lewes, East Sussex BN7 1XU, England
Distributed in Australia by NewSouth Books
University of New South Wales, Sydney, NSW 2052, Australia

For information about custom editions, special sales, and premium and corporate purchases,
please contact Sterling Special Sales at 800-805-5489 or specialsales@sterlingpublishing.com.

Manufactured in Canada

2 4 6 8 10 9 7 5 3 1

sterlingpublishing.com

Cover design by Elizabeth Mihaltse Lindy

IMAGE CREDITS: iStock: comotomo: 149; Shutterstock: Eisfrei: cover, 92, 109;
Reinke Fox: 138, 140, 142, 144, 148, 151; Christos Georghiou: 136, 137, 141, 145, 150;
imaginasty: cover, 128, 133; Alona K: 72, 86, 118, 127, 152, 172, 180; Le Panda: cover, 9, 10, 11, 15, 110;
mimibubu: 152, 192; Benjavisa Ruangvaree: vi, 134; Gorbash Varvara: cover, ii, 16, 20, 71, 186

Contents

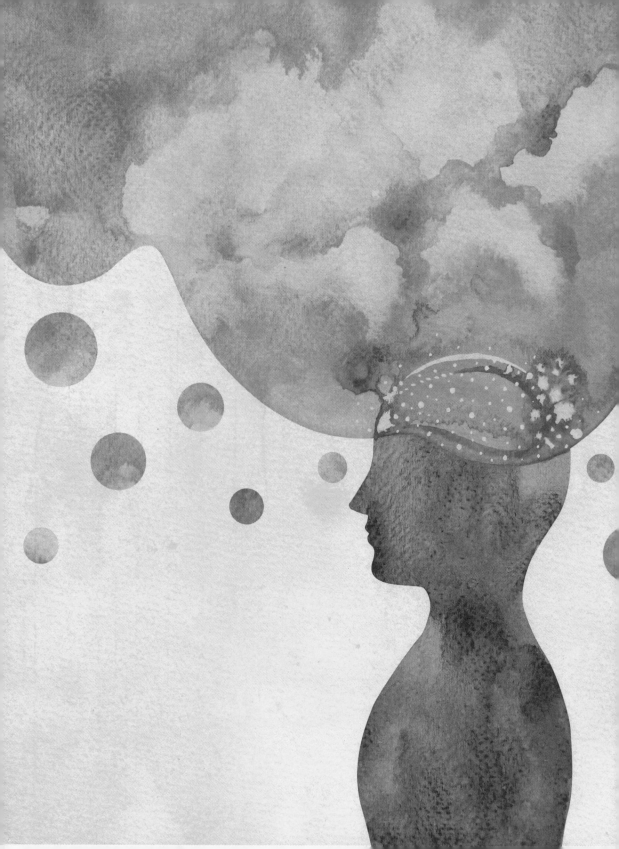

Introduction

The twenty-first century is the Age of Energy. Yet as the nations of the world race to develop the best sources of renewable energy for vehicles, homes, and industry, most of their people grow ever more weary. Technological achievements will be useless unless we also develop our ability to renew the energy in our own bodies, minds, and spirits as we confront this time of constant stimulation, information overload, and too much to do with far too little time in which to do it.

We have entered not only a new age but also what we call the "Now Age," a time when everything seems like it has to be done *now*!

As spiritual counselors with decades of experience using the psychological language that is astrology in our advising people from all walks of life, we can tell you that lately almost everyone seems to be suffering their own version of burnout. Far too many people are exhausted yet unable to sleep and too disheartened at perceived "failures" to do what must be done to achieve reasonable goals.

After decades devoted to pursuing the most effective techniques for living a life of quality, health, and meaning—and along the way developing many of our own techniques—we've written *Astrology for Wellness* to share what works for us, as well as simple yet effective techniques for developing and increasing an inner power supply. Our program has helped our clients to reclaim their personal power, heal, and rejuvenate.

We are not doctors, of course, and this book is not intended to be a substitute for the care and advice of any licensed practitioner you have researched and found to be someone whose advice you respect. We are, however, two people whose lives work well for ourselves, who are reasonably healthy and attractive for our ages, and whose dedication, life decisions, and energy levels have enabled us to produce a prodigious, sustained creative output over our more than forty happily married years together—output that could easily seem to be beyond what two people could produce in several lifetimes. It's a living. And an important part of our way of living is sharing our secrets for doing so with you.

We have crafted what we call "personality profiles" that can help you understand your unique traits so that you can incorporate our suggestions to create your own successful wellness habits.

The information in *Astrology for Wellness* is arranged so that it will first help you evaluate your strengths and weaknesses. Once you determine the vulnerable areas of your body, mind, and spirit, you can take measures to protect, nurture, and build them up.

We offer you tools, guidance, and energy exercises to create awareness, jump-start needed changes, and outline healing modalities, cell salt recommendations, aromatherapy, and lifestyle guidance that meet the personal needs of each Sun Sign.

Once again, we are not doctors, and you should not do anything or put anything into or even on your body before first asking your licensed physician about it. We are each unique beings and that uniqueness extends to what we are strengthened by, weakened by, and possibly allergic to, especially if we are already taking prescribed medications or even food supplements.

The useful practices in this book have helped us to lead a life of quality and meaning, and we are sharing them in the hope that they can help you, too, stay mindful and enjoy the journey on your own unique path. While wellness used to be confined to supplements, food, and fitness, these days the movement has expanded to embrace a more holistic vision of well-being that includes our emotional and spiritual health, not just our physical states.

As astrologers since the mid 1970s and authors of several internationally best-selling and influential metaphysical titles, we are delighted that the worldwide movement seeking optimum well-being now includes astrology. *Astrology for Wellness* contains simple, enjoyable—and what our many clients and we consider to be perceptive—tips that enable the reader to make small changes to their regimen and in their stream of both common and cosmic consciousness.

Our goal is that your mind, body, and spirit will feel renewed, preparing you to face the rest of your day without the extra burdens and worries that would otherwise deplete your vital energies. We believe that our spiritual energy is our core source of mental strength, and that tapping into that energy is the key to living a joyous, mindful, loving, and successful life. We have done it, and we know beyond doubt that you can do it!

We've packed these chapters with simple teachings that can produce powerful, life-changing results. We have learned many of these lessons from our years of astrological observations, personal readings, and psychic studies. *Astrology for Wellness* is our attempt to pass along information that has proven useful to us on the most practical level possible—teachings that have helped us to deal with life's inevitable problems, to enjoy life more, and to find health, love, and prosperity.

The practices in this book are like the pearl in the oyster, created and discovered as a reaction to the irritants we experienced. I, Monte, practiced astrology professionally when I gave up the musician's style of living after it threatened my health and marriage in 1981. This, the most difficult period in my life, put my metaphysical belief system to the strongest of tests. But I know now that these painful times, as well as the teenage years I spent poor and homeless, were also some of the most valuable experiences of my life. It was through facing and dealing with the many problems of these times that I saw daily proof of how astrological and metaphysical theories put into practice could actually have very positive, practical, physical results—even repairing what many might have thought irreparable. *Astrology for Wellness* is based on what we've lived through, studied, and practice.

One of the many fortunate results of my metaphysical investigations and practices was my being asked to take a job as a production assistant for a public television production in 1983. One job led to another, and soon I was a location scout and, on occasion, in charge of security and even a bodyguard working on feature films, TV shows, and commercials. My years in this fascinating business were made even more interesting by my advanced astrological knowledge. I was able to have astrologically oriented conversations filled with insights into the many interesting people, both famous and not so famous, with whom I worked closely. As I've often told my young clients, if you want to really have fun at parties and do well socially, don't learn the guitar like I did when I was your age, learn astrology and how to read tarot cards!

In between my movie jobs I devised a simple yet effective tool for using the wisdom of astrology for guidance. I am the author and inventor of *Karma Cards*, a unique astrology book/astrology flash-card package—a combination of astrology and tarot cards—that has helped hundreds of thousands of people around the world get in touch with the guidance available to them from their Higher Self at the same time as they are having fun. It has been in print continuously for thirty years and has been published in eighteen languages. I have received hundreds of emails from around the world thanking me for inventing a tool that helps people to help themselves by developing their own inner guidance system in such a pleasurable and interesting way. Many have shared their personal problems with me and asked for my advice. *Astrology for Wellness* is the "recipe" book I wished I could offer to each and every one of them as my answer. It's my way of sharing the good fortune I have enjoyed.

Devising systems for sharing the wisdom and knowledge that helps me succeed in life is also a way of reminding myself of what I too need to remember; because not only is my life as full of problems to be solved as anyone else's life, but also like everybody, sometimes I forget what I know truly works for me. That's why I have always believed, and will repeat many more times in this book, that just as our bodies need consistent, daily exercise to maintain themselves, we all need to exercise our belief systems, what we affirm to be true both with and without question, every day.

But examining, realizing, and experiencing what we believe to be true, though vitally important, is still basically a maintenance-level exercise program. To grow we must experiment. By investigating new ideas that appeal to us or those ideas that have helped others whom we trust and respect, we can discover whether these different ways of believing (be living!) can help us to be healthier, happier, and more successful—even in these most challenging times. Reading and taking to heart the teachings of some of the great sages, philosophers, and teachers of the past and present have helped Amy and me. When something sounded good to us, we tried it out. We knew when something worked because our lives felt better and we felt better about our lives.

Once you decide that there are things about your life that you desire to change, you have to be honest with yourself about fully examining what they are and the reasons you have allowed things to go on as they have. As the philosopher Gurdjieff said, "To get well we must first know we are sick." You can usually spot areas of your life that need changing because they are sources of pain, suffering, and sometimes, a good deal of boredom for you or for those who are close to you and who care about you. Things related to these areas don't seem to work well for you, no matter how hard you try. You may even be literally "sick and tired" from "beating your head against the wall." Words you say to yourself are powerful and have influence over your life.

Our pain can also be a spotlight shining on the areas of our life where our attention and our work are needed. And just like that spotlight, we are going to concentrate our light—the light of our awareness—on those painful areas because that is the kind of light that can heal them.

As you honestly confront those areas of your life that need work, it is very important that you take some of the responsibility for what has happened to you in the past. Taking responsibility for your life is an admission that you had the power to get where you are and, therefore, have power over what happens to you now and in the future.

For example, if your marriage has not gone well you cannot put all the responsibility for the situation on your spouse—even if it appears to be entirely your spouse's fault! My father was a New York City police sergeant and really saw it all. He warned me that many people told him that they had married their spouse expecting to be able to change them. These people married alcoholics, junkies, criminals, and other kinds of sick, often violent people. But as my father said, we can't change anybody else. It's hard enough to change ourselves—the only person we actually can change. Besides, putting all the blame on another person puts the situation totally in that person's control.

Similarly, if you have been unable to find a partner, you cannot blame your situation on the lack of "good," available members of the sexual orientation you desire to meet. Your actions and even your inactions, based on what you believe to be true about you and others, have resulted in your present situation and only you can fine-tune your beliefs until they produce the reality you desire to experience. I've seen miracles happen and the right partner appear as if from nowhere—but only when my clients were ready for that miracle to happen.

Today, usually under the banner of the much maligned and widely misunderstood New Age, there are many people who think that we each are totally responsible for the creation of every aspect of our own personal reality. I find this theory intriguing and worthy of further study, but I think an idea like that can be very confusing and even hurtful if taken literally at this stage of our development, especially regarding our being born into or otherwise experiencing circumstances that no reasonable person would ever have wanted to create.

The common denominator of all human-caused suffering is poor decision-making. That is how we truly create our reality and our future too.

Taking an honest look at yourself through the 5,000-year old lens of astrology can help you make better decisions. Astrology helped us to realize the things that we had brought upon ourselves as a result of our decisions and our beliefs and, equally important, how to work on them, using our strengths to compensate for our weaknesses, rather than worry about our having created situations that appeared to be well beyond the power of individual humans to create or even significantly influence.

And so we must look within and take notice of our inner dialogue, our astrological influences, and our reactions to and inactions regarding any and all situations. Where are we? What is the problem? What must be done to correct it? We must focus on the present moment because the present is the only place where our power is concentrated. The past is beyond our control and the future is . . . well, in the future. But we can affect the future by living and acting in the present moment. By feeling our power to control ourselves in the present moment we can extend that power to affect all areas of our experience. When our spiritual life force is strengthened, we feel more vibrant and can actually achieve a specifically desired shift or life change to our experience of wellness. It is our most sincere hope that sharing what works for us will help you identify and put into practice what works for you. We wish you love, light, and laughter—always and in all ways.

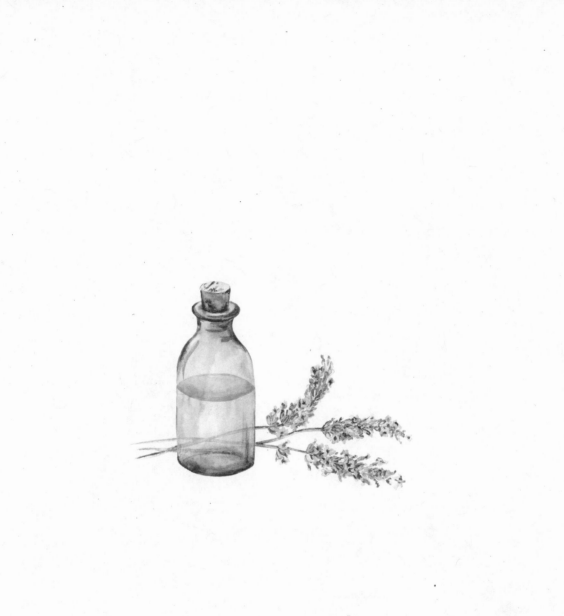

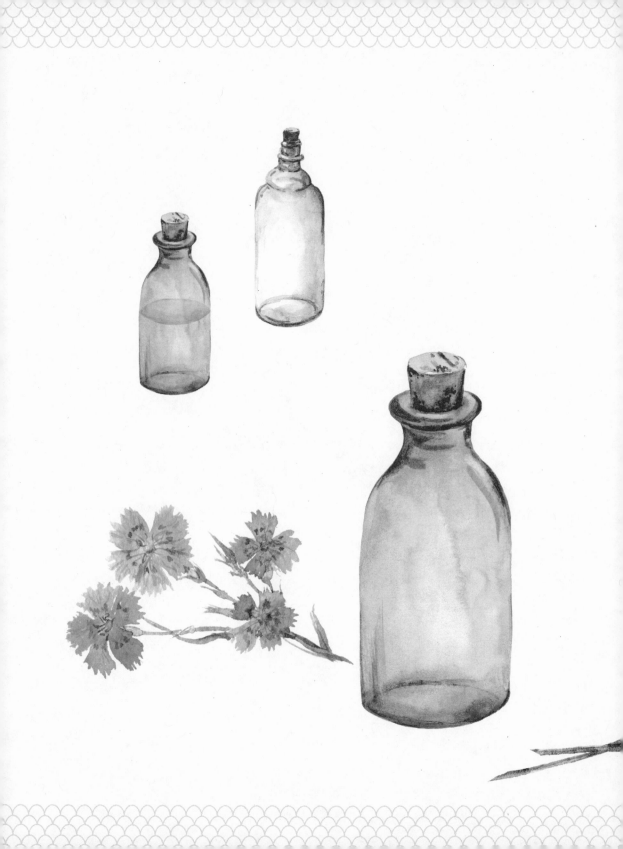

) 1 (

Some Notes

ABOUT

Wellness

We all want to live lives that are as healthy and happy as possible. It is obvious that some people are born with or become afflicted by serious health problems through no fault of their own, but it is equally obvious that many people have a part in creating the "dis-ease" that afflicts them.

In any case, we believe that it is just as important to well-being to stay balanced, to be mindful, and to avoid extremes in thinking and behavior as it is to drink plenty of pure water and eat nourishing, organically grown food. "Nothing in excess," is our motto. Being calm, open-minded, and flexible seems to help to stimulate our body's defenses and help with maintenance and even recovery. We are so used to our busy but peaceful lifestyle that we can actually feel disturbing energies flowing through us if we allow ourselves to be thrown off balance by toxic headlines and people. This book contains our favorite remedies for restoring ourselves and for better dealing with life's pressures and challenges.

One of the most important ones is, try to laugh, relax, and be conscious of your breathing when you have a "moment to breathe," another cliché that is a powerful use of words. Reach beyond accepted knowledge and remember that changing your life for the better is possible but only if you truly believe it is. If you don't, you'll self-sabotage. Talk to your body and tell it how much you love it. If this seems odd, think of how many times you've spoken to your car or some other inanimate object in which your consciousness did not reside! Loving your body is important because it's part and parcel of loving yourself the way you would love a child. Remember these ancient words (Matthew 18:3), "Lest ye be as little children, ye shall not enter the kingdom of Heaven."

As Hippocrates, the Greek physician referred to as the father of modern medicine and the author of the Hippocratic oath sworn by every physician, said, "Thy food shall be thy remedy." Today, we say that we are what we eat. In order to stay as healthy as we can, we need to eat healthy, natural foods that are as uncontaminated by pesticides and unsafe farming practices as we can obtain. I, Monte, have eaten this way since I was sixteen years old, and I consider it to be an important reason that I am reasonably healthy at sixty-eight.

If I ingest something that has chemical food additives, alcohol, or is otherwise adulterated, I can usually feel an immediate effect on my perception and, shortly thereafter, on my body. By eating the way we were intended to eat, we make it easier to think and plan clearly and react with emotional intelligence to the inevitable surprises and upsets of daily life, thereby helping us to make better decisions. Eating well is crucial if you desire wellness throughout a long and healthy life that is worth living. I have counseled extremely wealthy people who would trade their wealth for good health if it were possible. Always remember this when you are about to put your striving for wealth and "success" ahead of what you know to be best practices for optimum wellness.

It is a huge responsibility to counsel other people, but we have been extremely fortunate in the wise elders who have shared their secrets with us. One of them was the brilliant and legendary Professor Arnold Keyserling of the University of Vienna, whose teachings explored the shamanistic path designed to help each person find what the First Peoples around the world have called one's "medicine," that which heals us.

Down through the ages astrology has helped people to understand their nature and, in doing so, to explore natural remedies to help us heal. In fact, a conveniently forgotten fact is that Hippocrates taught that to properly treat a patient the physician should always know the patient's astrology chart!

If we are stressed and angry, however, or unable to fathom a way to cope with an apparently out-of-control life or victimized by others or harsh circumstances, then we cannot expect even the most perfect diet, the most thoroughly understood astrological principles or any other form of our medicine to keep us from becoming dis-eased. We believe, because we have seen it to be true so often, that if we are spiritually, emotionally, or mentally distressed, it is only a matter of time before this distress will trickle down into our bodies and manifest as a physical ailment.

In this book we share eight essential wellness practices for bringing balance to your inner and outer life, customized for each Sun Sign: empowerment, contemplation, relaxation, nourishment, intention, mindfulness, breathing, and good sleep.

Astrology for Wellness is chock full of metaphysical fitness tips for each Sun Sign. You'll have fun while identifying the core issues and areas where work needs to be done. And you'll be able to design a custom daily practice to produce actual changes in your inner emotional dialogue and daily healing habits that will produce seemingly magical changes in your life. We love to give our readers a renewed faith in achieving their goals, as well as giving actual suggestions for practical steps to succeed. Let's explore some new cosmic pathways to wellness, together!

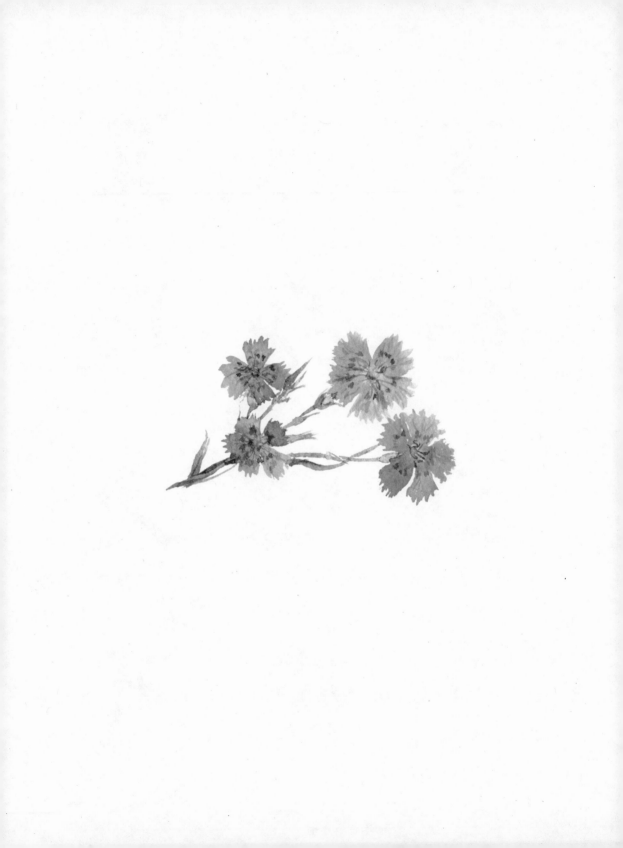

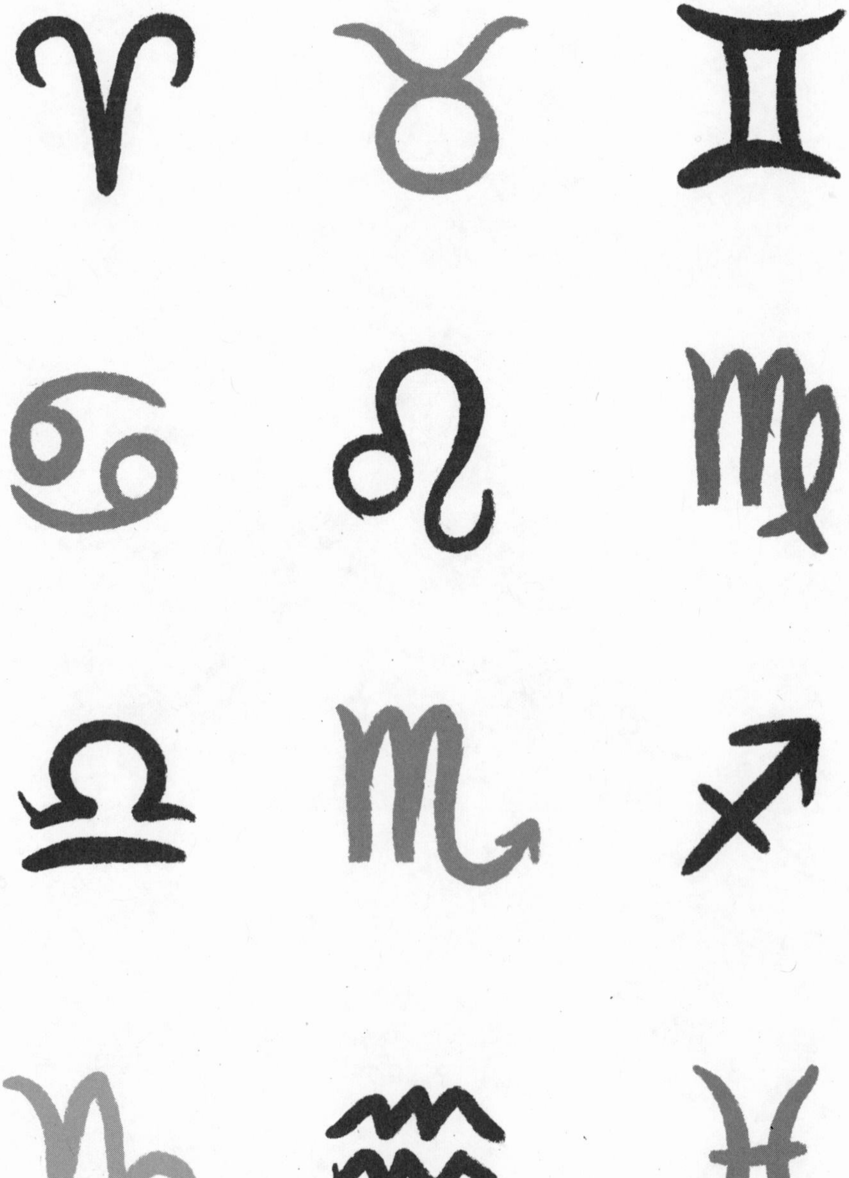

2

Astrology Works

—HERE'S HOW

It's all about gravitational waves. Whether or not you think astrology works, I hope you accept the fact that there is gravity. I thought so. I also assume you understand that gravity is an especially powerful force as it emanates from the large massive bodies we call *planets,* a word derived from the Greek word for *wanderer,* because the planets appeared to be stars that were not fixed in relation to each other but were slowly moving through the night sky as time passed.

Planetary gravity is so strong that the indescribably massive planets actually pull on and affect each other's orbit. In fact, the planet Neptune was detected before it was actually seen because astronomers noticed that another massive yet unseen and unknown planet-size body was influencing the orbit of Uranus.

So why should the jumble of gravitational waves emanating from the Sun, Moon, and all the planets, including the dwarf planet Pluto, have any kind of perceptible and—here's the kicker—predictable influence on us sentient beings here on planet Earth? And what about Earth, itself, pumping out its own gravitational waves that one might think would override the influence of the distant Moon, Sun, and planets? Earth's waves keep us attached to the surface of Earth, right? That's a pretty strong force and the extraterrestrial planetary waves affect us in ways that are subtle and occasionally, like in the case of a full moon, not so subtle (ask any police officer, EMT, or emergency room worker).

But how, I hear you asking, does astrology work? OK, I'll do more than tell you, I'll show you! You need two polarized lenses, like from polarized sunglasses, so if you wear them and don't feel like popping out the lenses and don't have another pair, get with a friend who also has a pair of polarized sunglasses.

Polarized sunglasses are so named because the lenses filter out all light waves that are not on what we will describe for this example as a "North Pole to South Pole" axis. If you take a polarized lens and then put a second one over it and rotate them slowly while looking through them, you will soon see that they do not let *any* light pass through them. This occurs when the polarized light axis of the two lenses forms a right angle. But how, you ask, does this example explain how astrology works? OK, the ground has been prepared, and here we go . . .

The Sun, Moon, and planets are bombarding Earth with gravitational energy waves that affect our planet's tides (the Moon) and weather (the Sun) and the same subtle but real planetary-orbit-affecting gravitational forces that enabled astronomers to discover the planet Neptune. When planets make various angles to each other, then these gravitational forces blend in ways similar to but more complex than in our polarized lens show-and-tell experiment.

These blended energies from the Sun, Moon, and planetary bodies are bombarding and having a perceptible influence on Earth and all beings. According to our view of astrology, we are, each of us, a living hologram of the energies that we ingested with our first breath the day we were born (Note: That is why caesarean births are accurate. In a perfect world, charts would be calculated by the time of a person's first breath and not "just" the equally miraculous passage from the mother's body into individualized personhood).

So astrology works because five thousand years of observing planetary interactions with daily life has enabled us to "read" the interaction between the various planetary wave energies in the sky today or at any given moment in the past or the future, and the hologram of our birth time that each of us carries within us. I realize that we are not our baby-self but I don't think I'm the only person who believes without question that with all of the changes I've gone through as a person, there is still a real and present part of me that has not changed that much since the day I was born.

One of my own astrological personality traits is to be quite skeptical, and if my research had not shown me the accuracy of what I am able to glean from a person's astrology chart, then I would not have wasted another minute on it. As it happened, when I met Amy in 1974 she was studying astrology and I was studying Amy, and so I learned astrology, and both events changed my life spectacularly for the better. Together, we have used astrology as a significant part of our language of love. *Astrology for Wellness* is the fruit of our years together and we are both humbled by our good fortune and are honored to share with you what has worked so well for us.

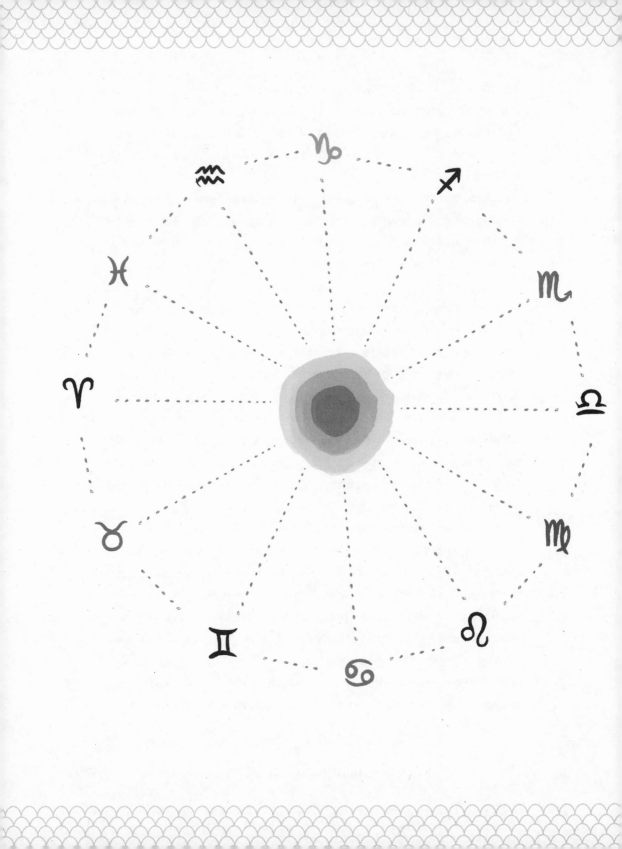

3

Your Sun Sign

PERSONALITY

Profile

Remember, all of the traits of the various Sun Signs exist in each "native" of that Sun Sign as *potential* traits to be learned about and explored mentally, physically, and spiritually. They don't just naturally arise in the full-blown way that they do when someone dedicates him or herself to self-improvement. No one is born as a pure manifestation of her or his Sun Sign. Life is all about learning and growth, and astrology helps in that process.

We like to think of astrology as the spice of life, but that metaphor also reminds us of astrology's limitations: one cannot survive by only eating spices. Taking the proper approach to astrology, i.e., it is a guidebook for exploring your potential, can lead to the optimum level of wellness possible to each of us.

An Important Note: The start and end dates for the twelve signs of the Zodiac are approximate, a fact that most astrology books fail to notify you about, because the day of the month when the Sun enters the various signs of the zodiac can change from year to year. Check the date of the sign change for the specific year of your birth to make sure which sign you truly are.

aries

MARCH 21–APRIL 19

PLANET: Mars—symbol of the energy available to the ego to get what it wants

ELEMENT: Fire—symbol of energy, action, and creativity

QUALITY: Cardinal—goal oriented, concerned with initiating projects or being enterprising

QUICK READ: Arians are cardinal fire. They know how to initiate action, how to push and work toward furthering their goals. They cannot wait to do what they have in mind to do. Therefore, patience is one of the most important lessons for Aries to learn.

COLORS: red (all shades)

PERSONAL QUALITIES: honest, brave, and headstrong

KEY WORDS: initiation • challenge • adventure • exploration • daring • courage • honesty • competition • innocence • action • aggression • spontaneity • discovery • creativity

ARIES NATIVES
ARE LEARNING ABOUT THE BEST
PRACTICES AND PITFALLS OF THE
FOLLOWING CHARACTERISTICS:

» How to be a self-reliant, independent thinker and doer

» How to command, displaying strength in such a way as to not simply appear bossy

» How to disagree with others without compromising convictions and opinions or fighting

» How to be a person to whom responsibility is an honor and not a burden

» How to be optimistic and resolute while endeavoring to do it your way

» How to best channel an innate competitiveness without alienating others

» How to balance a willful and total focus on goals with patience about their coming to fruition

◇◇◇◇◇◇◇◇◇◇◇◇◇◇◇◇◇◇◇◇◇◇◇◇◇◇◇◇◇◇◇◇◇◇◇◇◇◇

Aries

Those who aggressively strive to be pioneers in some way display the forceful, independent personality of the sign Aries. They act on their first impulse without any forethought and thrive when they are in charge of a project or working alone.

Aries is considered the first sign of the zodiac. Arians, as those born under the sign of Aries are called, can seem aggressive and forceful because they are trying to be independent. They like to be pioneers in some way, the first to do something. They want to do things in an original way. Even the way they are original can sometimes defy categorization. If anyone can spontaneously create a new way to be a pioneer, it is an Aries. They certainly don't like to be second or even to wait for anything for very long. They function best when they act on their first impulse and don't second-guess themselves. They hate lies and liars and can sometimes be too honest for their own good.

The symbol for Aries is the headstrong Ram. Each spring the desire to mate and stake his claim to his territory drives the Ram to display his bravery by butting heads with his competitors. After a few times, the one who can handle the headache and hasn't given up is the winner. People born under the sign of Aries share a lot in common with their symbol, the Ram. They are willing to butt heads with those they think are standing in their way. Sometimes, they will give up if they do not get their own way quickly enough.

The reason why Arians are sometimes not as brave, original, and pioneering as they wish they were is because people do not arrive in the world already an expert in the things their Sun Sign is known for. They have come into this world with the challenge of the astrological sign Aries because they want to learn how to accomplish something that has never been done before and accomplish it without letting fear stand in their way.

The lesson for Arians is that they must learn the hardest part of how to be brave. No Arian wants to think that they are letting fear stop them. However, because Arians are learning what it takes to be an uncompromising individual, they are, in effect, learning all the various aspects of what it means to be brave. Arians are more afraid of being afraid than they are afraid of any actual person, situation, or thing. This is the central challenge for all born under the sign Aries and it is also why they sometimes suffer from panic attacks.

They must keep in mind that any fears or self-doubts that are triggered in them are not signs of weakness or losing control or a guarantee of failure. They must not let fear of feeling any signs of fear in themselves paralyze them into inaction and even more self-doubt.

At their most basic level, our fears are a means of preventing us from getting hurt physically, emotionally, and financially. Fear is meant to keep us from repeating mistakes and to keep us out of harm's way. It is as natural an emotion as love; in fact, they are opposites. Negative fears are those that are irrational and counterproductive. They exist to challenge us into developing methods for coping with them. When we do, the memory of our negative fears enables us to see how strong we have become. Arians could not prove their strength to themselves unless they first became aware of their fears and then learned to deal with them. I purposefully do not say *overcome* or *eliminate* when it comes to fear. As a natural emotion, fear will always be with us. Fear is not a sign of weakness, but giving in to fears is.

Remember: Arians are LEARNING TO BE BRAVE.

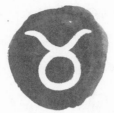

taurus

APRIL 20–MAY 20

PLANET: Venus—how we define and utilize beauty and attract our desires to us

ELEMENT: Earth—symbol of what you can touch, substance, practicality, and grounding

QUALITY: Fixed—stubborn, concerned with dependability, determination, and stability

QUICK READ: Taureans are fixed earth. They know how to sustain an effort in matters that concern talent, security, values, and finances. They do not like to quit, even when they should. Therefore, learning how to let go is one of the most important lessons for Taurus.

COLORS: spring green, blue, pink

PERSONAL QUALITIES: loyal, pragmatic, good-humored, reliable, and musical

KEY WORDS: slow • steady • values • money • caution • control • security • tenacity • texture • beauty • habits • supplies • kindness • calmness • romance • sensuality

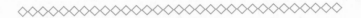

TAURUS NATIVES
ARE LEARNING ABOUT THE BEST PRACTICES AND PITFALLS OF THE FOLLOWING CHARACTERISTICS:

» How to plan your course of action before even the most minor undertaking

» How to be proud of your strength, persistence, and endurance and not just results

» How to make a secure, comfortable, and beautiful home for yourself and others

» How to live well by one's own definition and not that of others

» How to rely on your own memory and not be swayed by that of others

» How to truly appreciate beautifully designed apparel, jewelry, and fine dining

» How to appreciate music and singing, which you immerse yourself in totally and may actually participate in performing or creating

Taurus

Those who can cope with anything that gets in their way display the determined, steady, and methodical personality of the sign Taurus. They can be depended on to follow every step of a plan stubbornly and deliberately, especially when they know their reward will be pleasure and luxury.

Many people born under the sign of Taurus share a lot in common with their symbol, the Bull. Though they are usually patient and gentle, when pushed too far, Taureans can become like a bull tormented by a toreador's cape. Angry or not, they are so set on their goal that they can see little or nothing else. In fact, they sometimes think they must be equally set on the way they will accomplish their mission.

Many people born under the sign of Taurus are a source of mystery and awe to their friends because no one except a Taurus will exert the energy necessary to put up with a situation most other signs would just walk away from. But Taureans don't even like to walk around a situation, let alone walk away from one. Meeting challenging situations requiring patience and endurance is how they prove their abilities to themselves and those around them.

Taureans get the material comforts they need and overcome obstacles by exerting their immense power in a sustained and methodical manner, no matter who or what tries to make them give up on their efforts or even deviate from their plan. They function best when they are able to concentrate and stick to a preconceived plan.

The reason why Taureans are sometimes not as determined, patient, and comfortably well-off as they wish they were is because people do not arrive in the world already an expert in the things their Sun Sign is known for. They have come into this world with the challenge of the astrological sign Taurus because they want to learn how to be determined, patient, comfortably well-off or wealthy and how to cope with everything those things require.

If Taureans really wants to possess what they desire, they must learn to include in their plan to achieve their goal at least some room for flexibility and change because sometimes the best way to get what they want is to modify and adjust their plan of attack to the circumstances in which they find themselves. It is not enough to be a stubborn bull if you want to be a successful one.

Fear is the cause of Taurus's stubbornly clinging to a plan, a belief, or even a person when all the evidence points to the fact that it would be best to change that plan and belief or not see that person anymore. The fear of being proved weak and wrong and to have wasted one's precious time is the obvious cause. There is also the fear of having to face the unpredictable unknown and go through the struggle of coming up with a new plan, finding a new person, and having to learn a whole new way to proceed that is often strong enough to cause a Taurean to stay when they should go and to fight on when they should move on.

Taureans are, by nature, very resistant to listening to any advice that they think is not in agreement with the plan they have already decided on. What good is advice if a person has already decided that what they believe to be the way is the only way? As the English writer John Heywood said in 1546, "There are none so blind as those who will not see." You do not have to make big changes, but you do have to be open to change. Remember, change is the evidence of the existence of life.

Unswerving loyalty and devotion to those you love are among your most conspicuous traits if you were born when the Sun was in this sign. Also, you are conscious of every step toward prosperity, and you regard financial affluence as one of your highest goals. This attitude is prompted by the fact that the sign Taurus rules wealth.

Remember: Taureans are LEARNING TO BE STRONG AND RESOLUTE.

gemini

MAY 21–JUNE 20

PLANET: Mercury—how we use our logical mind

ELEMENT: Air—symbol of ideas, intellect, and communication

QUALITY: Mutable—flexible, concerned with adapting and blending

QUICK READ: Geminis are mutable air. They know how to adjust and improvise their style of communication to deal with fluctuations. Geminis can adapt themselves to their environment. Therefore, learning how to craft a unique set of core beliefs is one of the most important lessons for Gemini.

COLORS: white, yellow, multicolored patterns

PERSONAL QUALITIES: witty, changeable, versatile, talkative, well-read

KEY WORDS: duality • social skills • communication • mischief • cleverness • logic • restlessness • gossip • versatility • curiosity • precocity • duality • advertising • quick wit

GEMINI NATIVES ARE LEARNING ABOUT THE BEST PRACTICES AND PITFALLS OF THE FOLLOWING CHARACTERISTICS:

» How to be a multitasker and to work on several jobs or even careers simultaneously

» How to use your communication skills to inform others when your opinions are so changeable

» How to apply what you know to real world situations, turn talk into practical actions

» How to relate to others so they will allow you to be who you are

» How to see all sides of any argument and diplomatically change sides in a heartbeat

» How to experience the realization that your intellect usually controls your emotions

» How to accept that despite your voracious consumption of information, you cannot know everything about anything

» How to avoid negative consequences from a sometimes irrational fear of boredom

◇◇

Gemini

Those who are skilled at doing two or more things at the same time display the versatile personality of the sign Gemini. Their desire to comprehend and communicate everything quickly produces both an endless curiosity and an ability to take every side of an issue.

Those born under the sign Gemini are among the best communicators of information, especially things that they have heard and their opinions. Most of them do not gossip more than most people, they are just better at it and enjoy it more. You can bet that when a Gemini tells you something, it is the most up-to-date information available.

Yet, though they speak clearly and put their point across, they are often misunderstood. Most people want to be known for their unwavering commitment to a bunch of opinions regarding what is true about life. In fact, most people think that is what everyone has to do to function in the world, but Geminis do not think that way. They are curious to know what life is, and they are more than willing to adjust their beliefs when information that appeals to them comes along.

They want to experience life in as many different ways as they can. They may even go so far as to have something of a double life. At the very least, they have two opinions about everything—more if they have actually studied a particular subject in depth. They will do practically anything to avoid being bored, which, to a Gemini, is almost a fate worse than death.

Because they are interested in everything, Geminis become skilled at anything they put their lightning-quick minds to. They are also the most versatile of signs. It is a rare Gemini that only does one thing extremely well. They also have great dexterity.

Geminis do not just have two or three opinions; it is like they are two or three different people, and that has to be accepted by those who want to be close to them. Their changeability can be annoying or interesting, depending on how much you want people to be the same every time you see them. Geminis too, are the same every time you see them: equally changeable. As the saying goes, "It takes all kinds," and that includes the changeable Geminis we all know and love.

Geminis love to be up on the latest things and they try their best to know something about everything. This is the origin of stories about their legendary curiosity. Geminis think that if they only had the time and access to enough information, they could actually come to know everything. Nobody can give the appearance of knowing everything better than a Gemini. Though sometimes, they may find themselves arguing the exact opposite position of the one they held yesterday. This is a source of their charm. They also provide the rest of us a valuable service by reminding us not to be so certain that our truth is the only truth.

People who are just getting to know a Gemini may try to pin her or him down and consequently they may think that their new Gemini friend changes his or her mind too much. This is just how it appears on the surface. Geminis do not actually change their minds so much as they actually have two minds. Many thousand years ago, the ancient sages were wise to pick as the symbol for Gemini a pair of twins. For it is as if within them there are actually two different people with two different sets of values and opinions—maybe more. In fact, Geminis are legendary for functioning best when they have two or more things to do at the same time.

However, the lesson for Geminis to learn is that there is an important reason why they are not as knowledgeable quick, versatile, and skillful as they wish they were. They have come into this world with the astrological sign Gemini because they want to learn everything, especially how to be quick, versatile, skillful, and smart!

Remember: Geminis are LEARNING ABOUT LEARNING.

cancer

JUNE 21–JULY 22

PLANET: Moon—our emotional intelligence

ELEMENT: Water—symbol of emotion, intuition, and empathy

QUALITY: Cardinal—goal oriented, concerned with initiating projects or being enterprising

QUICK READ: Cancers are cardinal water. They know how to give and nurture as well as how to understand emotional processes. They can share feelings and be protective. Therefore, learning how to avoid being overprotective is one of the most important lessons for Cancer.

COLORS: silver, mauve, smoke gray

PERSONAL QUALITIES: caring, tenacious, sensitive, nurturing, and practical

KEY WORDS: clairvoyant • protective • heredity • emotions • moods • feelings • intuitions • reflect • respond • adapt • habits • cycles • motherhood • unconditional love • our past

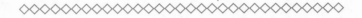

CANCER NATIVES
ARE LEARNING ABOUT THE BEST
PRACTICES AND PITFALLS OF THE
FOLLOWING CHARACTERISTICS:

» How to balance their respect for family and tradition with the need to change with the times

» How to accept the fact that they can forgive without ever forgetting

» How to be compassionate, even empathetic, without upsetting their sensitive stomach

» How to experience their tender, affectionate, and emotional nature while being self-protective

» How to see the tendencies and motivations of others without trying to "fix" them

» How to create secure circumstances for others and not feel incomplete when they "leave the nest"

» How to cherish and protect sentimental objects without becoming overly attached to them

Cancer

Those who can forgive the childish transgressions of those they care for display the nurturing, protective, maternal personality of the sign Cancer. They are shyly aware of their own past and can easily apply its lessons to create security in their daily life.

Those born under the astrological sign Cancer are well known for their ability to nurture others. They are especially sensitive to the ways people communicate their feelings and can be easily upset when there are bad feelings agitating those they care about. In fact, learning about feelings and the moods they produce are an important part of being a Cancer. In astrology, the Moon is considered a planet and associated with the sign Cancer. The Moon's ever-changing shape and its effect on the constantly shifting ocean tides is like our ever-changing moods, though the Moon's shape is a lot more predictable.

The past is very important to Cancerians. Their family history is especially so, either as a source of pride or as a painful experience affecting them as if it just happened. Either way, they will always want to relate what is going on in the present moment to something they have known in the past. By sticking with what is familiar or relating the new to what they already feel familiar with, they are able to feel secure. The symbol for Cancer is the crab. Feeling insecure makes them want to withdraw into their own version of a crab's protective shell.

The reason why Cancerians are sometimes not as secure, sensitive, and nurturing as they wish they were is because people do not arrive in the world already an expert in the things their Sun Sign is known for. They have come into this world with the challenge of the astrological sign Cancer because they want to learn how to be secure, sensitive, and nurturing. Cancerians are legendary for their ability to nurture people and projects along, for they sense the needs of others on an emotional level. However, it is important that they remember that meeting their own emotional needs is just as important. Often, they have to be able to nurture themselves, for they are so good at nurturing others that others forget how Cancerians too need nurturing.

When they feel emotionally secure there is no one who is more giving then a Cancer. However, when they feel emotionally insecure, they are totally unable to give and this can confuse those who have come to depend on them. Being shy, especially at those vulnerable times, Cancerians would be reluctant to tell anyone of their needs for fear that those who they care for would let them down. A Cancerian would be able to forgive a person who was unable to be there for them at a critical time, but they would never forget what had happened.

Cancerians are often affected by the time of day they decide to do something. Plans made at night become harder to make real in the daytime, and vice versa. If they find themselves forgetting to put the plans of the previous night into practice the next day, they must be as patient and forgiving of themselves as they would be with the mistakes made by a child learning and growing.

Before anyone can help others, they have to feel secure. The first rule of warfare is "make your base secure." Without a good foundation, no home will last very long. Cancerians would do well to remember that they may not be as strong as those around them think they are, but they are certainly strong enough to do what has to be done to make their dreams come true. They must resist withdrawing into their shell if they start to feel insecure. Their usual courage, patience, and gentle energy are more than they will need to make of their life what they will.

Remember: Cancers are LEARNING TO BE NURTURING.

leo

JULY 23-AUGUST 22

PLANET: Sun—our ego and our sense of purpose

ELEMENT: Fire—symbol of energy, action, and creativity

QUALITY: Fixed—stubborn, concerned with dependability, determination, and stability

QUICK READ: Leos are fixed fire. They know how to persevere and be respected by becoming a steady and focused creative force. They like to lead and be noticed. Therefore, learning that true leadership is doing what is best for those you lead is one of the most important lessons for Leo

COLORS: gold, orange, yellow

PERSONAL QUALITIES: creative, dramatic, proud, organized, and romantic

KEY WORDS: self-assertion • creativity • recognition • theatricality • hobbies • leadership • love • pleasure • fun • hospitality • openheartedness • appreciation • playfulness • entertainment

◇◇◇◇◇◇◇◇◇◇◇◇◇◇◇◇◇◇◇◇◇◇◇◇◇◇◇◇◇◇

LEO NATIVES
ARE LEARNING ABOUT THE BEST
PRACTICES AND PITFALLS OF THE
FOLLOWING CHARACTERISTICS:

» How to command attention, respect, and loyalty, especially in group endeavors

» How to craft and present a unique, impressive, and noble presence

» How to show others how to live life to the fullest, especially when romance is concerned

» How to be as sincere, honorable, and reliable as possible in light of political realities

» How to use humor, generosity, and forgiveness as both the right and most practical tools

» How to balance being devoted to those you care about with your own human needs

» How to honor and enjoy each moment, including the ones that demand drudgework

◇◇◇◇◇◇◇◇◇◇◇◇◇◇◇◇◇◇◇◇◇◇◇◇◇◇◇◇◇◇

Leo

Those who enjoy creating solutions and being leaders display the self-expression and confident personality of the sign Leo. They are romantic, generous with their affections, and proud to acknowledge accomplishments.

Leo is the sign of the creative organizers of the zodiac. Practically no one is as good as they are at recognizing the solution to a problem and organizing the means to solve it. It is this ability that gives rise to Leo's reputation as a great leader. Like all leaders, most Leos feel more comfortable when they are delegating what has to be done rather than taking care of the routine details themselves. They get annoyed with themselves for this trait, but not for long, because Leos like themselves a lot. They put themselves where there is much that needs to be done, and they associate themselves with the right group of people so that their creative input is always welcome, even if they are do not always jump in and get their hands dirty.

The symbol for Leo is the strong and proud male lion, a most appropriate symbol. Not only is a group of lions referred to as a "pride" of lions, but also the importance of personal pride to those born during the time of Leo cannot be overstated. They would not want to be connected to anyone or anything that they did not feel was up to their high personal standards. Their pride inclines Leos to provide those born under the other signs of the zodiac with a good example.

Showing us all how things are done is a special gift possessed by Leos, which is why they have such a knack for drama. Their gift can be acting, the arts and music, or any form of display. Their generosity requires them to create situations and objects that will benefit and entertain them and those they consider worthy to be connected with them.

The lesson for Leos is that there is an important reason why they are not as proud, powerful, and good at leading as they wish they were. They have come into the world when the Sun was in the astrological sign Leo because they want to learn the best way possible to become the kind of powerful leader they can be proud to be. Sometimes, even the best of leaders must put on an act to get the job done.

Of course, when Leos are creating things for others to look at, their audience's feedback becomes very important to them. If their dramatic gestures are not acknowledged sufficiently, their pride will be hurt. Then they might forget their responsibilities to others and maybe even try to use their power to influence others in a dictatorial fashion.

Leos are legendary for their ability to help and protect those who acknowledge them as special people. They gain a sense of their own self-worth by giving what they think others need from them. However, it is important that they remember that they too need help and protection. Leos are usually too prideful to ask for help.

Leos' reputation for having a large ego comes from this inability to ask for help. When they put such obvious value on being supportive to others, yet don't ask for the same, it is easy for others to assume that Leos think they are either too good to ask for assistance or that they don't think anyone has the ability to help someone as great, strong, and talented as a Leo.

Many Leos do believe that anyone who needs help is weak and incapable of being a leader. However, we all need help. Like the lion and other kings, Leos should get used to letting those who care about their welfare bring them gifts for a change. No one knows how to live as royally as Leos do. When they learn how to accept help and to delegate their authority, then they can show the world how to really live the good life.

Remember: Leos are LEARNING TO BE PROUD LEADERS (and how to get people to follow them!).

virgo

AUGUST 23–SEPTEMBER 22

PLANET: Mercury—how we use our logical mind

ELEMENT: Earth—symbol of substance, practicality, and grounding

QUALITY: Mutable—flexible, concerned with adapting and blending

QUICK READ: Virgos are mutable earth. They know how to be of service and how to review, fix, edit, and adjust to circumstances. Virgos can be critical and analytical. Therefore, learning how to be mindful of their perfectionism is one of the most important lessons for Virgo.

COLORS: navy blue, gray, green, tan

PERSONAL QUALITIES: analytical, discreet, practical, intelligent, and detail oriented

KEY WORDS: energy • thought • observation • study • discernment • division into component parts • criticism • reason • logic • connection • adaptation • health

VIRGO NATIVES ARE LEARNING ABOUT THE BEST PRACTICES AND PITFALLS OF THE FOLLOWING CHARACTERISTICS:

» How to use their analytical ability without a susceptibility to worry and perfectionism

» How to develop healthy habits of eating, dressing, and personal grooming

» How to be practical and address fears that can lead to impracticality

» How to not let self-doubt and self-criticism work against their ambitious nature

» How to use their notable sense of humor to relieve anxiety in themselves and others

» How to criticize themselves and others without appearing harsh or pedantic

» How to keep the desire to do things correctly from resulting in procrastination

Virgo

Those who are driven to perform useful acts to the best of their abilities display the skillful, hardworking, and humble personality of the sign Virgo. Their close attention to the smallest of details is matched by their ability to analyze people, things, and systems.

Virgo is the astrological sign associated with the myriad details of life. Virgos like to get things done. It is as if they are driven to perform useful acts to the best of their ability at all times, no matter how big or small the task. Virgos are very careful and methodical in everything they do because they value order and neatness. When involved with people or situations that are messy or disorganized, they will probably find themselves irritable and unable to apply themselves to the task at hand in their customarily efficient manner.

The symbol for Virgo is a young, virginal woman. She represents the value Virgos place on purity of mind and body. In a way, they are always young, trying to learn all they can, and learning the way a young person would.

Developing their skill and confidence in themselves as hardworking people is more important to them than the praise of the crowd. However, they are not machines and Virgos do need some thoughtful words of encouragement from those with whom they work and work for. A pat on their back and appreciation for a job well done will usually satisfy them more than fame or money.

The lesson for Virgos to learn is that there is an important reason why they are not as useful, skillful, and perfect as they wish they were. They have come into this world with the astrological sign Virgo because they want to learn the best way possible to be useful and skillful and the best person that they can be. Not perfect, but the best that they can be.

Many Virgos do not realize they are perfectionists of the highest order. Why? Because they feel that if they really were perfectionists, they would be much more closer to perfection than they are! That goes to show what perfectionists Virgos can be.

The lesson for Virgos also involves the sign's legendary tendency to over-analyze and worry about things. Worry is actually a combination of two fears resulting from the very process of analysis. To analyze anything you have to know as much as you can about it. However, to analyze a living person or an ongoing situation you are never going to have all the information you would like to have. The first fear that produces worry is that you do not have enough information to fully understand a situation. The second fear is that you will not be able to deal with the consequences of a situation unless you fully understand it and can predict what is going to happen.

Virgos must avoid letting their tendency to worry about how things are going to turn out influence them too strongly. They have to suspend their tendency to criticize what they experience, no matter what that is, and hold it up to some impossible standard of perfection.

If they really want to be as practical as most Virgos would like to be, then they must realize that they will use their gift for criticism in a construc-tive way, by waiting to use it until they have first listened to and absorbed the information they receive. They must stay out of their own way and not let their tendency to focus on some minor imperfection prevent them from hearing another part of their message that proves to be the key to help them unlock the door to life's glorious bounty.

Remember: Virgos are LEARNING HOW TO ATTEND TO THE DETAILS.

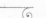

libra

SEPTEMBER 23–OCTOBER 22

PLANET: Venus—how we define and utilize beauty

ELEMENT: Air—symbol of ideas, intellect, and communication

QUALITY: Cardinal—goal oriented, concerned with initiating projects or being enterprising

QUICK READ: Libras are cardinal air. They know how to be fair in relationships and will work for justice. They can be diplomatic as well as surprisingly aggressive. Therefore, learning how to attain a balanced, harmonious approach to life is one of the most important lessons for Libra.

COLORS: light blue, royal blue, pastels

PERSONAL QUALITIES: artistic, refined, poised, intelligent, and tactful

KEY WORDS: partnership • union • sophistication • good taste • yin and yang • balance • cooperation • fairness • quality control • aesthetics • harmony • romance • opinions • diplomacy

LIBRA NATIVES
ARE LEARNING ABOUT THE BEST
PRACTICES AND PITFALLS OF THE
FOLLOWING CHARACTERISTICS:

» How to keep the desire for a balanced approach from leading to indecisiveness

» How to function alone if necessary as an essential ingredient for healthy partnerships

» How to balance fairness with the practical necessities of dealing with others

» How the definitions of art and beauty mean different things to each person

» How to relate to human foibles in the preparation for and execution of partnerships

» How to remain calm and persevere even when events are inharmonious or threatening

» How to fight for peace, love, and justice

Libra

Those whose goal is the resolution of conflict through compromise display the refined and diplomatic personality of the sign Libra. They constantly strive to balance the scales of justice, regarding legal decisions and committed partnerships of all kinds.

Libra is the only sign whose symbol is not a living being. Its symbol is the old-fashioned balance scale, the symbol of equal measure and justice. The time of Libra is, in the Northern Hemisphere, when the harvest is brought in, weighed and measured for sale, against other years, and other farmers. Perhaps this is why Libras are such an interesting mixture of refined judgment and fierce competitiveness.

Libras are very partner-oriented and often find it difficult to function efficiently without one. It's not that they depend upon their partner for much. Libras need a partner so they can find out what they themselves think about something by bouncing it off of another person. When they find a partner who, in this way, enables them to feel the way they want to feel, they seek to make the partnership permanent. This often leads to partnerships that others have difficulty understanding. It also makes Libras very concerned with living up to the conditions of partnerships. This is the origin of contracts and the law itself and explains why Libras are often found in professions concerned with ensuring the correctness of people's behavior.

Librans will work very hard to attain the goal of resolving conflict, either through compromise and diplomacy or by fighting the good fight if they are forced to. They are constantly trying to balance the scales of justice regarding practically everything, and that can be very trying, not only on themselves but also on those around them. Their desire to make the perfect decision can sometimes prevent them from acting decisively until it is too late to do so.

The lesson for all Libras to learn is that there is an important reason why their judgment is not as refined, elegant, and accurate as they would like it to be. They have come into this world with the astrological sign Libra because they want to learn how to develop their judgment and become the best competitor for the finer things in life. Libras hate anything they consider not up to their standards and only want to be surrounded by the best.

Librans too often allow themselves to be persuaded to abandon their own judgments and distrust their intuitions. It is like they allow the scales to be put out of balance just because they cannot believe they have arrived at a perfect solution, a solution coming from within themselves. Many Librans are constantly seeking advice, but then they waver uncertainly between an instinctive faith in their own opinions and a fear that disaster awaits them unless they follow the advice of someone else. If they lose confidence in their own views and try to reconcile them with what others may think, they can become confused, vulnerable, and aggressive.

Librans must avoid letting their tendency to look for the equal correctness of the opposite of what they are being told influence them too strongly. They will gain no points for coming up with an argument to the information being offered. This is not a contest between what they think and what this book says. They have to suspend their tendency to argue with what they are being told.

The scales that symbolize Libra are a nonhuman device intended to indicate the relative weight or value of everything by attaining a position of rest, resolution, and harmony. A scale never brought to a state of equilibrium is almost worthless. Librans have a natural affinity with the unseen, intuitive side of life. With the exceedingly rare and keen perception characteristic of the sign Libra, no human attainment is beyond their grasp.

Remember: Libras are LEARNING HOW TO BE FAIR AND BALANCED.

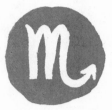

scorpio

OCTOBER 23–NOVEMBER 21

PLANET: Pluto—how we deal with power and change

ELEMENT: Water—symbol of emotion, intuition, and empathy

QUALITY: Fixed—stubborn, concerned with dependability, determination, and stability

QUICK READ: Scorpios are fixed water. They know how to understand what motivates them and what makes others tick. They are devoted to exploring life at its extreme boundaries. Therefore, learning how to function well with less passionate people is one of the most important lessons for Scorpio.

COLORS: black, dark red, maroon

PERSONAL QUALITIES: intense, obsessive, loyal, determined, and passionate

KEY WORDS: investigation • conscience • secrets • magical • psychology• precision • mysteries • good detective • transformation • power • legacy • sex • regeneration

SCORPIO NATIVES ARE LEARNING ABOUT THE BEST PRACTICES AND PITFALLS OF THE FOLLOWING CHARACTERISTICS:

» How to accumulate and use personal power to effect change in all areas

» How to keep secrets

» How to persevere in the face of opposition without using unjust or self-destructive methods

» How to be passionate

» How to experience the magical side of life, especially as it relates to sexuality

» How to balance their fascination with the natures of reality, death, and transformation with daily life

» How to be intense in a world where most people are reluctant to display or encounter intensity

Scorpio

Those who are compelled to know the secrets of power and control display the magnetic and investigative personality of the sign Scorpio. They are so passionately interested in living life to the fullest that they often find themselves involved in extremely intense situations.

Scorpio is the master detective of the zodiac. If there's something or someone Scorpios wants to know about, there is nothing or no one who can prevent them from discovering the hidden truth. It is as if they feel compelled to know all the secrets just in case they need to use them to prove how powerful they are.

When it comes to their own secrets, Scorpios are equally skilled at keeping them from others. In this way they prevent others from having power over them. They will rarely volunteer information for the same reason. Power in all its forms is one of the biggest issues for Scorpios to deal with. Most of them are powerful and know it.

However, if Scorpios doubt their own power, they become so attracted to proving that power that they are willing to do practically anything to do so. This can obviously put them in intense situations. Scorpios usually keep their feelings and thoughts to themselves, for they are too deep for mere words. However, they will not hesitate to make the perfect comment at the perfect time, especially if it will deflate someone's pompous ego. Scorpios aspire to a level of purity that is hard for the other signs to even imagine. This is why they are more than willing to set straight everyone whose deeds do not measure up to their words. Scorpios are keen students of psychology and always want to know what makes people do the things they do.

Compulsions and strange behavior of all kinds do not faze a Scorpio one bit. In fact, their curiosity is piqued. In undeveloped Scorpios there is a tendency to use their intimate understanding of human motivations for ruthless manipulation cunningly designed to attain selfish goals. However, most Scorpios are as fearless as their most well-known symbol, the scorpion. But like a scorpion, they can be so intent on stinging something that they end up stinging themselves. Scorpios are often misunderstood because of the intensity of their passion. The forceful way they communicate their truth is such that people can't believe that they really mean what they are saying.

Scorpio is the only sign that has other, lesser-known symbols. The two we find most important to further understanding the sign's meaning are the eagle and the snake. The eagle flies higher than any bird and the snake is the creature lowest to the ground. This is because Scorpio is associated with the extremes of the both the highest and the lowest existing at the same time. For example, Scorpio is the sign associated with sexual reproduction, a function that is accomplished using organs of the body also used for elimination of its liquid waste products.

The lesson for Scorpios to learn is that there is an important reason why their life does not provide them with as many peak experiences as they would like. They have come into this world with the astrological sign Scorpio because they want to learn how to develop their ability to work their powerful will on the world. The sign Scorpio rules magic and they want to make big changes in their lives, the kinds that appear to other people as almost magical transformations.

When Scorpios focus their energies on controlling others, they find in the end that it is they themselves who end up being under the control of others. However, when they turn their efforts toward self-control, the influence they have on both others and the world around them seems to be without bounds. It is as if the best way for them to control a situation is to be in control of themselves.

Remember: Scorpios are LEARNING HOW TO BE POWERFUL.

sagittarius

NOVEMBER 22–DECEMBER 21

PLANET: Jupiter—how we deal with success

ELEMENT: Fire—symbol of energy, action, and creativity

QUALITY: Mutable—flexible, concerned with adapting and blending

QUICK READ: Sagittarians are mutable fire. They explore the world in every way so that they can discover universal truths and share them. Therefore, learning where and when not to speak their truth is one of the most important lessons for Sagittarius.

COLORS: rust, purple (all shades)

PERSONAL QUALITIES: generous, cosmopolitan, humorous, optimistic, well-traveled, and honest to a fault

KEY WORDS: freedom • theories • teaching • learning • world travel • philosophy • expansion • nature • increase • encouragement • prosperity • jovial • positive outlook • luck

SAGITTARIUS NATIVES ARE LEARNING ABOUT THE BEST PRACTICES AND PITFALLS OF THE FOLLOWING CHARACTERISTICS:

» How to balance their desire to be totally moral and ethical with daily life's challenges

» How to show good will by accurately gauging who is ready, willing, and able to hear the truth

» How to make a living fully actualizing one's philosophy

» How to remain open, tolerant, and considerate even when being so is not fashionable

» How to be kind, friendly, and loyal to those who deserve such treatment, yet who disagree with one's philosophy

» How to keep from imposing strongly held beliefs on those with other ideas

» How to be philanthropic, sharing wealth of all kinds, including intellectual and spiritual wisdom

Sagittarius

Those who seek to share all the knowledge and wisdom they encounter display the philosophical and broad-minded personality of the sign Sagittarius. They are not afraid to interact with those quite different from themselves if such interaction results in an expansion of their understanding of the world.

The symbol for Sagittarius is Chiron, the bow-wielding Centaur—half-man and half-horse. Chiron the Centaur was the first doctor of herbal medicine and a wise sage. In Greek mythology, he was the teacher of the great warrior Achilles.

The legend of Chiron may have started out with stories of a wise and skillful hunter, perhaps the leader of the first tribe to hunt from the back of a horse. The other tribes might have seen them as being half-man and half-horse. Travel on horseback made it possible for people to see many different places and tribes with all kinds of unique customs. When they returned from their journeys, they kept their own tribe hypnotized with stories of these far off lands.

Those born under the sign of Sagittarius share this love of travel, animals—especially horses—the great outdoors, natural healing, and all things foreign. They are the philosopher-teachers of the zodiac, and without this vital function, each generation would be forced to start from scratch without the accumulated wisdom of the ages to guide them. Sagittarians seek out knowledge and the wisdom to use it properly. They are interested only in the ultimate truth because, otherwise, less than the ultimate would not be worth knowing and teaching to others.

This is why Sagittarians have such a reputation for being blunt. Sagittarians feel that anyone who is telling the truth should be able to defend their position against any question, even if their question is totally tactless and without regard for social customs. Sagittarians are in a hurry and want to keep traveling, learning, and spreading what they've learned. They don't have time to waste. Never expect them to apologize for having annoyed someone when they were only trying to get at the truth.

The lesson for Sagittarians to learn is that there is an important reason why life does not provide them with as many opportunities to travel, to learn, and to teach, as they would like. They have come into the world with the astrological sign Sagittarius because they want to learn how to study, how to travel, and especially, how to teach. They can use their desire and capacity to expand their understanding of the way the world works to take them around the world, both through travel and through travel in their mind via philosophy and learning. Publishing, social media, and broadcasting are ways to bring their world, what they have learned and believe to be true, to us.

When Sagittarians are required to act immediately, without having the time to think about what they are doing, they possess all the courage they need to do anything they need to do. However, when they are allowed the luxury of having enough time to think about what is required of them, they are inclined to be timid and cautious. It is important that Sagittarians not become so inspired by each new piece of wisdom they learn that they decide to put off the plans of yesterday to make yet another grand plan to change their life, and then cancel their plans tomorrow when new information becomes available.

It is also important that Sagittarians avoid their tendency to resist taking care of the details necessary to implement any successful plan. No sign is as fearless and broad-minded as they are when it comes to encountering the new and the strange, yet they need to develop tolerance for the necessary and the routine. Thinking big is a useful trait, but it will only take you so far.

Remember: Sagittarians are LEARNING HOW TO BE OPEN-MINDED.

capricorn
DECEMBER 22–JANUARY 19

PLANET: Saturn—how we deal with restrictions

ELEMENT: Earth—symbol of substance, practicality, and grounding

QUALITY: Cardinal—goal oriented, concerned with initiating projects or being enterprising

QUICK READ: Capricorns are cardinal earth. They know how to be disciplined in matters of resources and goal planning. They take action based on practical needs and the desire to be respected by those they respect. Therefore, learning how to deal with authority is one of the most important lessons for Capricorns.

COLORS: black, dark brown, gray

PERSONAL QUALITIES: ambitious, prudent, self-disciplined, thrifty, and traditional

KEY WORDS: permanence • tradition • conservation • organization • responsibility • realism • definition and understanding of rules and limits • test of time • authority • concern

CAPRICORN NATIVES
ARE LEARNING ABOUT THE BEST
PRACTICES AND PITFALLS OF THE
FOLLOWING CHARACTERISTICS:

» How to balance being logical, serious, and conservative with deeply felt emotional needs

» How to be respectful and punctual in a world in which these traits are not always appreciated

» How to use all available assets, including people, to further ambitions

» How to interact with, attain, and maintain authority

» How to define and attain true success

» How to laugh at the darker aspects of being a human to manage fears

» How to conserve resources and get the job done in the most efficient manner

Capricorn

Those who are willing to do what is expected of them in order to reach the pinnacle of success display the conservative and practical personality of the sign Capricorn. Their persistence and ability to focus on a goal enables them to become figures of authority.

A mountain goat with a fish's tail symbolizes Capricorn. A curious symbol, to be sure, but yet it perfectly represents the dual nature of those born during the time of Capricorn. The mountain goat is tireless as it makes its way to the top of mountain after mountain. Most Capricorns are equally tireless in their efforts to get to the top of their respective profession. Most people might think that Capricorns desire above all to attain fame and the respect of the masses. It is more accurate to say that they most crave the respect of those that they themselves respect. This is as important to them as is living in wealth and style, yet another way they gain the respect of the "in crowd."

To get to the top, Capricorns are willing to do what is expected of them. This gets them the reputation of being conservative, when deep inside, they are quite sensual. They are conservative in the best sense of the word. You conserve what you have so that you will have enough when you need it. This is true practicality. Capricorns make wonderful executives. In fact, it is difficult for them to show their true worth until they are left alone to assume some kind of definite responsibility. Once they feel this weight resting on their shoulders they will rise to the occasion, succeeding when others would fail. Once they realize that making something of themselves is up to them, they display a kind of energy that can overcome almost any obstacle.

Remember the fish's tail that the Capricorn mountain goat is dragging behind him? The ancients used the element water to symbolize emotion, and the tail is used by fish to propel and steer themselves in their watery world. Capricorn people have very deep and real emotional needs that can slow them down considerably or even stop them in their tracks.

The lesson for Capricorns centers on the important reason why their life does not provide them with as many opportunities to enjoy success, wealth, and happiness, as they would like. They have come into this world with the astrological sign Capricorn because they want to learn the best way to achieve success, wealth, and happiness! They know in their heart that there are actual techniques they need to learn and lessons they need to apply in their life before they can attain their full potential.

Their awareness of how far they have to go to achieve the respect they crave can sometimes get to them and make them pessimistic or, less often, depressed. This tendency actually comes not from the realization of how far they have to go but from the fact that they will rarely allow themselves to become inspired and energized by what they have already accomplished. Though they may not see it as well as those around them, they have, from a young age, already accomplished many things that would be sufficient to delight those who are not Capricorns. Further contributing to their tendency toward depression are the pressures caused by their desire to maintain a prosperous appearance, keeping pace with both fashion and tradition, while at the same time living in luxury and ease and, in some way, above the level of the masses whose praises they seek.

When Capricorns start on the road to success, their persistence and their ability to focus on a goal enable them to succeed and to become authority figures in their chosen field. If they can do what has to be done and maintain a sense of humor to help them get through the difficult times, they are unstoppable.

Remember: Capricorns are LEARNING ABOUT AUTHORITY.

aquarius

JANUARY 20–FEBRUARY 18

PLANET: Uranus—how we keep life fresh and exciting

ELEMENT: Air—symbol of ideas, intellect, and communication

QUALITY: Fixed—stubborn, concerned with dependability, determination, and stability

QUICK READ: Aquarians are fixed air. They know how to be friendly as a way to have people accept their original and somewhat radical ideas about how to benefit humanity. Therefore, learning how to preserve what is worth keeping while innovating new ways of doing things is one of the most important lessons for Aquarius.

COLORS: electric blue, sky blue, ultraviolet

PERSONAL QUALITIES: unique, brilliant, inventive, articulate, and progressive

KEY WORDS: humanitarian • inventive • detached • radical • altruistic • rebellious • scientific • eclectic • genius • eccentric • alternative • original • futuristic • history buff

AQUARIUS NATIVES
ARE LEARNING ABOUT THE BEST
PRACTICES AND PITFALLS OF THE
FOLLOWING CHARACTERISTICS:

»   How to be friendly and good natured even with people who seem to be causing problems rather than solving them

»   How to discern what must change and what is worth keeping

»   How to communicate forward-thinking concepts to those not used to such ideas

»   How to feel free yet be a productive member of society

»   How to innovate ideas that are imaginative and inventive and not constrained in any way

»   How to inspire confidence in others while not feeling required to conform to their expectations

»   How to stay current with the ideas of fellow thought leaders while endeavoring to leap ahead

◇◇◇◇◇◇◇◇◇◇◇◇◇◇◇◇◇◇◇◇◇◇◇◇◇◇◇◇◇◇◇◇◇

Aquarius

Those whose concern for the good of all impels them to invent solutions to society's problems display the humanitarian and free-thinking personality of the sign Aquarius. They learn from the past to affect the present so it will become the future they envision.

The symbol of the sign Aquarius is the Water Bearer pouring out his bounty to quench the thirst of world. For this reason, many people mistakenly think Aquarius is a water sign. Water was the element the ancient sages connected with the realm of emotion, empathy, and intuition. However, Aquarius is not a water sign. The element associated with Aquarius is air, the realm of ideas. People born under the sign Aquarius like to think in broad and theoretical terms and they want to "pour out" their ideas to quench the thirst of the world.

Being mistaken for a water sign is a very significant clue to the lesson for Aquarians. Water symbolizes emotions and empathy, and Aquarians are often perceived to be lacking in both. Aquarians are the mad scientists and absentminded professors of the zodiac. They require freethinking minds, unfettered by tradition or fear of disturbing the status quo. Aquarians detest linear thinking and are quite comfortable jumping from one idea to another until they surprise everyone around them by coming up with a workable plan for improvement of the matter at hand or a brand new invention.

The emotional detachment necessary to clearly see society's problems and to try to solve those problems without regard to the ramifications of the actions necessary to make these sometimes drastic changes make Aquarians seem to lack empathy for the hardships of individuals. Aquarians should examine actions they plan to take to make sure their well-intentioned actions will not be hurtful to others.

Once the scientific mind of an Aquarian is finished thinking about a subject theoretically, the Aquarian returns to the world of emotions. In fact, they are not comfortable with strong emotions in themselves or in others and can easily feel themselves being overcome by feelings of empathy for those less fortunate. This is what inspires them in the first place to come up with solutions to society's urgent problems.

Babies do not arrive in the world already experts in the things their astrological signs are known for. Aquarians are here to learn how to invent a way to make real the future they can so easily see in their mind's eye! This is the reason why their life does not provide them with as many opportunities to enjoy the freedom and other resources necessary to turn their innovative ideas into reality as they would like.

When Aquarians finally become convinced that they must stop dreaming about the kind of future they would like to live in and start working to make it a reality, they can be counted on to work until their goals are achieved. In fact, they sometimes make such extreme changes that in their enthusiasm to get rid of the old ways they can destroy valuable things from the past that still have great usefulness. The old expression for this is, "Throwing out the baby with the bathwater."

If Aquarians want to have the kind of life they have always dreamed of having, they must avoid letting their tendency to go to extremes cause them to imagine that they must make radical changes in their life that are really too much to ask of themselves and others—changes that are bound to be too difficult to maintain. People do not usually have to make sweeping, radical changes in their life to bring in the love, wealth, and success that they desire, especially the kind of extreme changes that an Aquarian would be willing to make without a second thought.

Remember: Aquarians are LEARNING HOW TO BE DIFFERENT AND MAKE A DIFFERENCE.

pisces
FEBRUARY 19-MARCH 20

PLANET: Neptune—our capacity for compassion and self-sacrifice

ELEMENT: Water—symbol of emotion, intuition, and empathy

QUALITY: Mutable—flexible, concerned with adapting and blending

QUICK READ: Pisceans are mutable water. They know how to shift, merge, and change and be highly sensitive and empathetic to the emotional needs of others. Therefore, learning to keep their sense of self while helping others is one of the most important lessons for Pisces.

COLORS: lavender, sea green, aqua

PERSONAL QUALITIES: empathetic, artistic, compassionate, selfless, and psychically attuned

KEY WORDS: sensitivity • spiritualism • receptivity • moodiness • caring • intuition • otherworldliness • inspiration • faith • idealism • fantasy • imagination

◇◇

PISCES NATIVES
ARE LEARNING ABOUT THE BEST
PRACTICES AND PITFALLS OF THE
FOLLOWING CHARACTERISTICS:

» How to be compassionate without undue self-sacrifice

» How to live in this world while believing in and working
to create a better world

» How to merge with the infinite through good works,
prayer, religious fervor, or meditation

» How to receive empathic and ever telepathic
information without the loss of personal identity

» How to organize others in philanthropic endeavors

» How to merge a basically idealistic nature and tendency
to daydream with real world needs

◇◇

Pisces

Those whose concern for the good of all compels them to become emotionally involved with those in need display the empathetic and compassionate personality of the sign Pisces. They can see and feel the interconnectedness of all things on an intuitive and psychic level.

Pisces is the last sign of the zodiac. Because it is the last of the twelve signs, it contains a bit of all of them. This is one explanation of why Pisces people are so easily able to understand how other people are feeling. In fact, Pisceans are so sensitive to the feelings of others that it is not good for them to be near people who are angry, sad, or disturbed. Sometimes, it is hard for those born during the time of Pisces to understand why they are feeling the way they are. If they take the time to investigate a little, they often realize that they are literally picking up on the feelings of others.

Pisces is associated with both empathy and telepathy. This natural ability to be invisibly connected to those around them and those around the world is both the blessing and the curse of all Pisceans. It enables them to feel exactly how to help those they care about, which is a Piscean specialty. It also exhausting and hard on a Piscean person's emotions to have other people's lives intrude so on their own.

Sometimes, naturally, there is a strong desire to escape from doing the double duty of experiencing both their own emotions and the emotions of those around them. This is why Pisceans often develop a means to escape from their sensitivity. No sign is as good at creating their own fantasy world, either through writing, dance, acting, and the visual arts, through mood-altering substances, or through making enough money to make their world as isolated and comfortable as possible. They get into trouble when they use drugs, alcohol, sex, gambling, religious zealotry, or any other escape devices that overwhelm their common sense and senses and block out the real world.

When they turn their sensitivity to the real world, Pisceans have the capacity to make incredible amounts of money in business ventures. If you think that seems unlikely given Pisces' reputation for dreaminess and escapism, remember that as the last sign with a bit of all the other ones. They have the ability to achieve an overview of any business situation and their sensitivity to others enables them to know how others will feel and act. That enables them to make accurate predictions that tell them how to act to reap the greatest rewards.

The lesson for Pisces centers on the important reason why their life does not provide them with as many opportunities to use their unique sensitivity to others to gain the appreciation and respect of those they would most like to help and associate with. They have come into this world born under the astrological sign Pisces because they want to learn how to get close enough to people to be of assistance to them without becoming overwhelmed by their needs and actions.

The more honest and honorable Pisceans are, the more they hesitate. They seem to fear that they may not be able to fulfill their promises or that the world will expect more of them than they can give.

Pisceans are most aware of both the things that unite us all and the immense differences between people. This is one of their great strengths, but if they let themselves be totally ruled by their emotions or let the sorrow of the human condition push them to escapist behavior, their great strength can turn into a great weakness. When they learn to balance their innate intuitive skills with a logical approach that does not ignore what is real but unpleasant, they can accomplish great things.

Remember: Pisces are LEARNING HOW TO BE CONNECTED TO ALL.

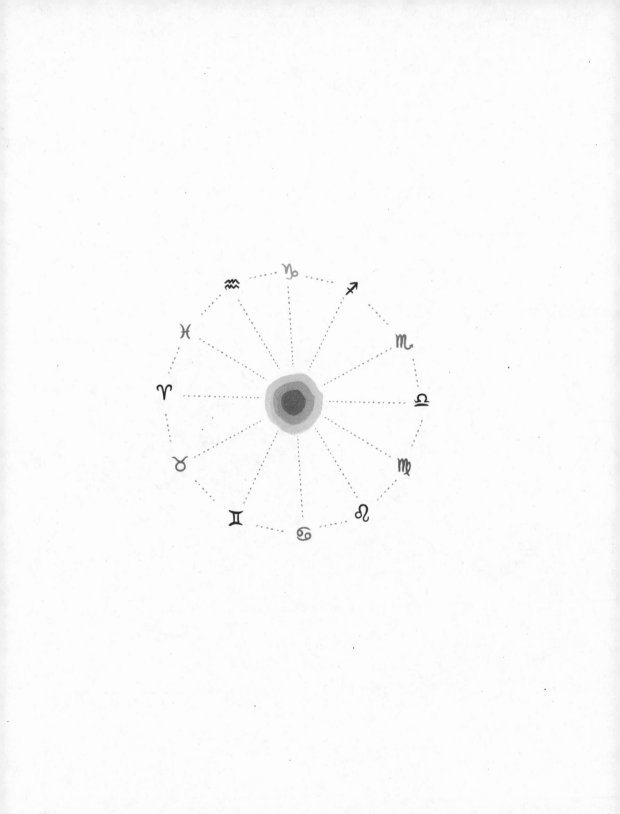

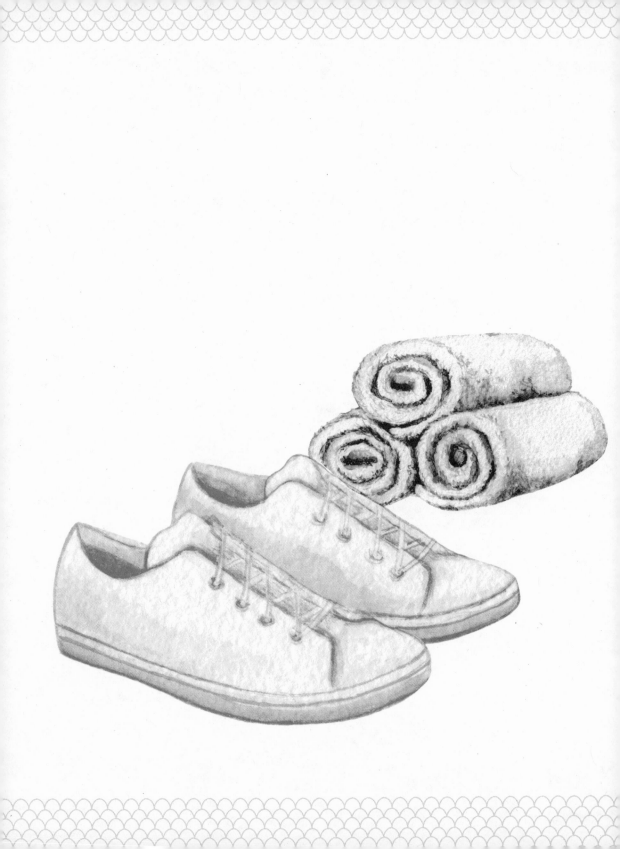

4

Wellness &
Fitness Tips

FOR

Each Sign

Running on the treadmill may work for some people, and Pilates appeals to others. Each sign is associated with a different part of the body. Each has its own strengths and weaknesses. The trick is finding a wellness plan and a workout style that matches your astrological personality and lifestyle.

aries

MARCH 21–APRIL 19

In astrology, Aries rules the head and the face. What's going on in an Arian's head—especially feelings of stress caused by feeling afraid or humiliated, missed deadlines, and lost opportunities—strongly influences what is going on in the body and makes Aries prone to headaches, toothaches, and neuralgia around the jaws.

Arians can burn out from too much work more easily than other signs. They're so busy, they haven't got time to be sick, but when they do fall ill, they usually make a speedy recovery but can lose their vaunted optimism if the recovery takes too long. Arians need to be careful of doing things too quickly, as they may injure themselves with knives, scissors, or metallic objects with sharp edges.

They should take care not to strain their eyes. Little "time outs" are good for an Aries: hot baths, five minutes in a hammock, getting their hair done—these will work wonders to heal and rejuvenate.

Aries likes to work out fast and furiously and usually alone. Interval training and its micro bursts of very high-intensity exercise coupled with short durations of timed recovery can work well for them. Even so, Aries needs to be careful of doing things too quickly.

Because Aries rules the head, sometimes headaches can make working out unadvisable. Aries is the sign of pioneers, so newly devised methods and long hikes in the fresh air will help clear their heads as well as heal, nurture, and rejuvenate their adventurous spirits.

Massage with a focus on the forehead and the temple area would be especially calming and helpful.

taurus

APRIL 20-MAY 20

Taureans usually enjoy good stamina throughout their lives, but when they do experience issues, the problems tend to occur in the sinus area, throat, and lungs. These parts of the body can be vulnerable and subject to repeated infections. Neck and voice problems are also common complaints, as the body part that Taurus rules is the neck.

Taureans tend to like sweet, creamy desserts, which can eventually lead to weight issues if eaten frequently or in excess. Fatty, high-calorie cuisine should be avoided. Taureans should also stay away from foods that are high in sodium or caffeine, as these can have a troublesome effect on their systems. Taurus loves the outdoors, so meditative time spent in beautiful gardens or arboretums would be a healthy habit to develop.

Taurus likes it slow but steady, so the treadmill works as does weight training for Taureans who like to prove how strong they are. Bulls need to make a plan and follow it faithfully, though they don't mind skipping a day here and there, especially if it's for a spa day or another luxurious experience.

Taureans must take care not to strain their necks when they exercise. They can also have issues around flexibility and would benefit from an unhurried, gentle yoga routine in a beautifully appointed studio. Stretching tense muscles can give pleasure and Taureans should never try to push themselves beyond that point.

Tactile Taurus knows how to get comfortable and relishes massages with a slow, even, steady pressure.

gemini

MAY 20-JUNE 20

Geminis need to be careful of health problems such as asthma, bronchitis, and the flu. This is because they tend to be intellectual, busy types who keep going even when overtired. They can become very run down, and their resistance is affected if they don't get enough rest. But they hate to be confined to bed!

They sometimes have a problem taking good care of themselves because they are constantly on the go and often forget to adhere to regular eating and sleeping schedules.

They must, therefore, try to establish a healthy routine and balance, which will reduce their erratic energy levels.

The symbol for this sign is the Twins, and it often seems that there are two personalities in each Gemini. Easily bored, Geminis should work out with several different friends and/or trainers.

Their best workout would be Pilates, which improves both flexibility and strength, or to vary their exercise regimen to include every method that interests them. Gemini rules the upper shoulders and arms, so chin-ups and pull-ups, even from a squat with feet never leaving the floor, work well.

Geminis tend to have sensitive nervous systems; therefore, whole body gentle massages with soothing music can calm their nerves. They are usually in hurry, so a hands-only massage will help them to stay focused and in the game when time is short.

cancer

JUNE 21-JULY 22

Cancerians are emotional types who may suffer from stomach problems and are prone to indigestion when under stress. They tend to bottle things up. As they do not like to burden other people with their problems, they tend to suffer in silence.

Typical Cancerians need material security, plenty of affection, and a sense that they are needed. As long as these needs are met, they can handle a lot. Wholesome food and regular meals are important to Cancer. Overindulgence in sweets, especially those they've enjoyed since childhood or that help them recall a happy time, can result in extra weight gain. Because theirs is a water sign, Cancerians should try taking long, warm baths to relax.

Cancer rules the past and the stomach area, so core training using old school methods like medicine balls, kettlebells, or sit-ups will help strengthen their midsection. Core work, especially Pilates training, is about will power, strength, and stabilization, all areas closely related to the sign's astrological affiliations.

Cancer is the sign of the home and the nurturer, so workouts should either be done at home or with partners chosen because they are like family or because they are less advanced and need the Cancer's guidance and encouragement.

A loving lymph massage will help detox, ease, and soothe a Cancer's melancholy moods or hurt feelings.

leo

JULY 23–AUGUST 22

Typical Leos are happy, healthy, energetic people as long as they feel loved and appreciated. If for some reason they are not getting the attention or affection that they crave, Leos will become dramatic and complain. As the "life of the party" they can sometimes overindulge in rich food and wine—too much of this will have repercussions.

Leos should take care of their hearts and backs, as these are the parts of the body that Leo rules. Whatever physical weaknesses they have, typical Leos will enjoy only a brief rest before recuperating vigor and being up and on the go again. To be out of commission for long is intolerable to a Leo.

Leo is the sign of the leader but also of the performer and so dance-oriented or martial arts workouts are perfect for keeping a Leo fit and looking like a star. Leos like to be allied with the most prestigious people, places, and things, so working out at home is a nonstarter.

Leos must avoid showing off when they exercise or they will find themselves out of the action quickly. It is rare to find a Leo without at least one story of an injury resulting from their attempt to impress someone.

Deep-pressure back massage will help relieve tension and transform a roaring lion into a purring kitten. Leos will benefit even more from massage if they can refrain from conversing with their massage therapist.

virgo

AUGUST 23-SEPTEMBER 22

Virgos are typically healthy and usually take good care of themselves. However, if terribly anxious or unhappy, they may succumb to their sign's tendency toward hypochondria. Virgos can experience frequent stomachaches stemming from their restless, nervous nature.

To maintain their health, they should be wary of working too much and instead learn to relax. However, Virgos often have to trick themselves into relaxing by thinking of it as one more job on their long to-do list. They should be aware of being overly critical, and do worry-releasing practices. The phrase, "no worries," repeated like a mantra and felt to be true, if only for a minute or two, can relax them quickly. Virgos should also avoid alcohol and foods that are very spicy.

Practical Virgos would benefit from functional fitness: short, intense sessions utilizing regular, everyday movements such as reaching, stooping, bending, or stair-climbing to improve focus, coordination, and strength.

Shutting down a Virgo's calculator of a brain requires that they work out in ways that pay attention to counting. Virgo rules the intestines, so they need to be strict with their pre-workout diet and avoid exercises that involve risks that cause worry.

A precise, organized, pressure-point massage would serve a Virgo well.

libra

SEPTEMBER 23-OCTOBER 22

Expecting a good life, Libras easily become forlorn whenever difficulties arise and can suffer from paralyzing indecision in their mental efforts to resolve problems. When Libras are unhappy, they tend to overeat in a misguided attempt to combat feelings of exhaustion, as if the wonderful food will instantly fuel them and get them back up to speed. They are happier and healthier when engaged in rewarding work. It can also take a great deal of effort for them to motivate themselves to exercise regularly.

Libras have a generally strong constitution, but their kidneys and bladder may let them down later in life due to their fondness for luxurious wining and dining.

A meditative, elegant exercise such as tai chi enhances a Libra's neuromuscular coordination, muscle isolation, and increased stability while improving their skill and posture. Libras are social, so they need a workout that allows them to see and be seen and even be heard, like skiing and the equally important après-ski time.

Anything involving balance is perfect for Libras, from skateboarding to TRX to boogie boards. Libra rules the kidneys so Libras need plenty of pure water to keep them working properly. Cranberry or cherry juice can help this process.

Deep tissue massages coupled with polarity work will also help a Libra stay balanced.

scorpio

OCTOBER 23–NOVEMBER 21

Scorpios are quite often physically strong and enjoy good health. Scorpio rules the eliminative and sexual organs. Scorpios need to release their stress and tension with lovemaking. Their passions run very deep and their emotional needs are great. Boxing, martial arts, archery, and shooting sports appeal to them.

Nose and throat problems, bladder disorders, and problems with the eliminative and reproductive organs are the most common Scorpio illnesses. Their health can suffer if their daily life is not conducive to helping them to feel safe and powerful in some way. It is easy for them to become debilitated if they constantly have to stay on the alert and defensive to a perceived threat.

People born under this sign benefit from taking antioxidants. Scorpios have amazing recuperative powers, and they are likely to recover speedily if they are ill. Their emotions run deep and their physical needs are great. Cycling, swimming, or water-resistance workouts would enhance the cardio fitness of a Scorpio to improve performance and stamina.

Scorpios can be extreme so extreme sports may attract the fittest among them. Tantric yoga and any workout related to their sexual prowess works. While sex is a good workout for all twelve signs, Scorpios refine it to an art form.

Sensual hot stone massages would be very healing for Scorpio.

sagittarius

NOVEMBER 22–DECEMBER 21

Adventurous, energetic, and active, Sagittarians fear being ill or confined. As they are so full of life, their energy levels fluctuate and often get depleted. They should watch out for excess weight around the hip and thigh areas, the parts of the body that Sagittarius rules.

Any kind of routine taxes the Sagittarian optimism. However, their positive, friendly outlook helps them to overcome setbacks quickly. Sagittarians tend to take physical risks, so accidents arising from sports can be expected from time to time. The jovial Jupiter influence can lead a Sagittarian into overindulgence in food or drink, especially those from places unfamiliar to their friends and family.

The fitness regimen of a Sagittarius should include some kind of training that is done outdoors. Sagittarians have the mindset of an adventurer. They do well when they include traveling to new locations, skiing in the Alps, kickboxing in Nepal, or trekking in nature in an exotic locale.

They might want to join a rock-climbing gym, a suitable alternative to a conventional strength-training regimen, which would be perfect for the Sagittarian's exploring nature. But they should be careful not to forget that nature can be unforgiving if reasonable precautions are not taken.

Massaging the hips, buttocks, and thighs will help restore the sense of free movement that a Sagittarius craves.

capricorn

DECEMBER 22-JANUARY 19

Capricorns need to learn to relax. Long periods of work and heavy responsibilities could lead to aches, stiffness, pain, and stress-related illnesses. Capricorns are acutely aware of the time and tenacity needed to accomplish their goals and need to be careful of depression, especially when they feel their process has hit a wall. They need to make sure to get enough rest at night and enough light during the day. Capricorns usually exercise only if it fits into their rigid work regime or will enhance their efforts at becoming respected by their peers and superiors.

Bones are likely to be their vulnerable body parts, especially knees and elbows. Their resistance to disease often increases with age. Capricorns get younger as they get older! They are usually moderate in their habits and because of this they often live to a ripe old age.

Capricorns like to set goals for themselves and make action plans. Weight-bearing exercises are beneficial to them in that they help to increase bone density. Range-of-motion exercises designed to maintain the movement and flexibility of joints should be done daily.

Earth-centered activities such as dog walking, gardening, raking, mowing the lawn, or digging the ground would also appeal. Capricorns like to stick to a routine.

Stretching massages with pain-relief lotions or herbal wraps would do wonders for their well-being.

aquarius

JANUARY 20-FEBRUARY 18

Aquarians have vast amounts of mental energy but often drive themselves into the ground, not knowing when they are tired. They have the habit of not listening to others' advice to slow down, and they can be rebellious patients who won't admit defeat. Aquarians need lots of fresh air, plenty of sleep, and regular exercise to stay healthy.

Often, their work puts great demands on their eyesight and their time, but they should never be so busy that they miss an appointment for an eye exam. They can have poor circulation, manifesting itself in leg and ankle problems, which are the body parts that Aquarius rules.

Aquarius is the sign associated with electricity, making it imperative that their exercise regimen be beneficial to their spine and nervous system. Wearable technology, such as wrist-based heart-rate monitors that have integrated performance-tracking systems, will motivate future-thinking Aquarians to supercharge their aerobic training sessions with an extra layer of biometric data.

Aquarians would be drawn to workouts that shock muscles, challenge weaknesses, and get them out of their comfort zone. They often choose equipment and exercises that many would deem unorthodox, odd, or just plain weird. Old school workouts coupled with those based on the latest theories about longevity would be the perfect combination for an Aquarian.

Massage with a special focus on ankles and calves will be especially beneficial and grounding to Aquarians who need to rest their minds as well as their bodies.

pisces

FEBRUARY 19–MARCH 20

Typical Pisceans are healthy people as long as they are either loved or have someone—or even a pet—that they love and can dedicate their lives to. Unhappy Pisceans are vulnerable to alcohol, drugs, or other ways of escaping reality, which is not good for their mental and physical health. Pisceans can worry and tend to develop insomnia. If they do relaxing forms of exercise or meditation, they can stay positive.

The constant effort of avoiding negativity is the cause of much distress to many Pisceans, who are so intuitive, they often know when someone else is ill and can feel their pain. Pisceans also need to take care of their feet, the part of the body that Pisces rules. They should always wear comfortable shoes.

Because Pisces rules the feet, an enjoyable movement-focused fitness routine, such as Zumba, ballroom dancing, or swing or salsa dancing accompanied by good music, is a perfect way to get a high-intensity workout.

Of course Pisces is the Fish, so swimming workouts enable this water sign to go with the flow and get fit. They should try swim drills to increase speed and endurance. And little impact means no sore feet! They should always make sure they are well-hydrated.

An impressionable Pisces will relish a reflexology foot massage, which addresses the energy points for all the organs in the body.

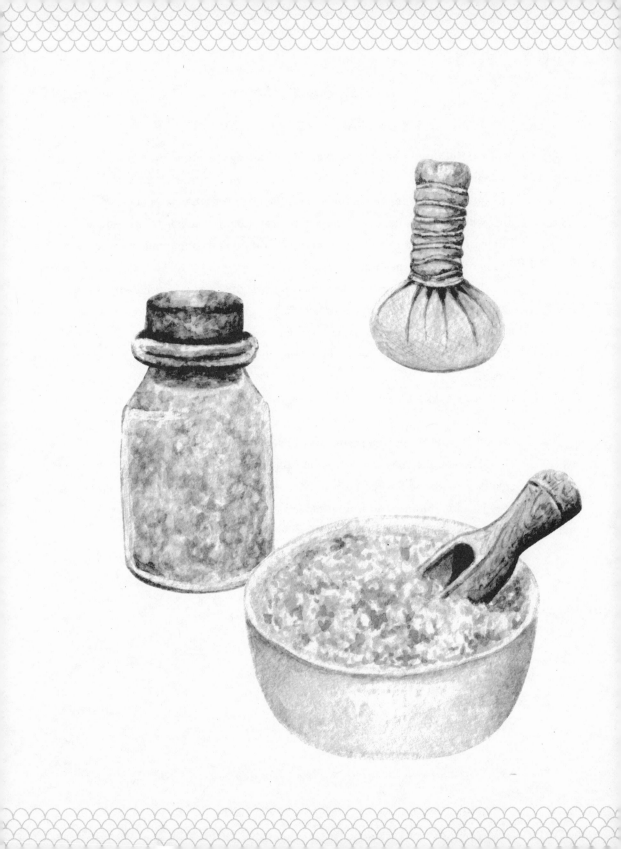

5

The
12 Cell Salts

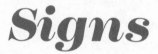

Signs

Hippocrates, the Greek physician, regarded astrology an essential piece of a physician's knowledge. It has been accepted practice in many cultures to consult the stars when choosing the best time for a medical procedure.

The association and use of cell salts and the zodiac is primarily based on the work of American physician George W. Carey and his partner, astrologer Inez Eudora Perry. Our friend the astrologer Leor Warner introduced Amy and me to this fascinating study in the 1970s.

The twelve cell salts are important for mineral balance and overall wellness. A good way to start to improve your body's mineral balance is by taking the cell salt associated with your sun sign.

Following is a description of the cell salts associated with each sign, along with the conditions and parts of the body they focus on.

ARIES

Aries governs the head, and so it governs the brain, head, face, eyes, and ears. Aries individuals are often willful, headstrong bosses with lots of ambition and drive. They have a tendency toward mental and physical burnout. Kali Phosphoricum (Cell Salt #6) nurtures the nerves and brain. It is used to help with side effects of stress and exhaustion: headaches, sleeplessness, crankiness, and poor memory.

TAURUS

Taureans are dependable, hard-working individuals who enjoy the arts: music, design, fashion. Viusalizing a bull, the symbol of Taurus, it isn't surprising that Taurus rules the throat, neck, larynx, tongue, and thyroid. Natrum Sulphuricum (Cell Salt #11) is the corresponding cell salt. It is a remedy for the flu virus and key to a healthy digestive system—all very important for overindulging Taureans.

GEMINI

Geminis love to communicate. Always on the move, they tend to overthink. Gemini rules the nervous system, hands, arms, shoulders, lungs, and ribs. Kali Muriaticum (cell salt #5) is Gemini's cell salt, responsible for helping the majority of body functions run more smoothly. It acts as a nerve tonic and helps relieve colds, coughs, sore throats, sinusitis, and bronchitis.

CANCER

Cancerians are hypersensitive, caring people who nurture others. They seek security and stability. This tenderness can cause them to be moody. Cancer governs the chest, stomach, womb, and pancreas. Its cell salt is Calcarea Fluorica (Cell Salt #1), which encourages toning of the cells and tissues, bones, muscles, teeth, and veins. Calc Fluor also combats fatigue, an important remedy for the sign that rules caregiving.

LEO

Leos are passionate, showy, and attract attention. They bask in love and appreciation. Health issues can develop when Leos feel disrespected or neglected. Leo rules the heart, upper back, blood, and spleen. Its cell salt is Magnesium Phosphate (Cell Salt #8). Mag Phos targets the heart. Mag Phos also treats sharp, nerve-related pain, cramps and spasms, headache, earache, and sciatica.

VIRGO

Virgo governs the sympathetic nervous system, colon, and small intestine. Virgos are detail-oriented problem-solvers with a practical work ethic, but their perfectionism can cause depletion from worry. Their cell salt is Kali Sulphuricum (Cell Salt #7), which supplies oxygen to the cells, and supports digestion. Kali Sulph also aids skin issues, yeast infections, and upset stomach.

LIBRA

Libra personalities value harmony, balance, and fairness. They are very social, work well in teams, and avoid taking sides. Libra rules the kidneys, lower back, and adrenal glands. Libra's cell salt is the pH balancer Natrum Phosphoricum (Cell Salt #10). Nat Phos is used for digestive issues, heartburn, GERD, and rheumatism as it balances acidic conditions of the cells and blood.

SCORPIO

Scorpios experience intense emotions. Scorpio governs the reproductive, urinary, and excretory organs. Its cell salt is Calcarea Sulphuricum (Cell Salt #3), which is an important cleanser and purifier helping the body dispose of stored waste and revitalizing the sex organs. Calc Sulph works to help eliminate infections, including colds, sinusitis, and some skin conditions.

SAGITTARIUS

Sagittarians are full of enthusiasm. They love sports and traveling and have big ambitions. Sagittarius rules the liver, thighs, hips, and pelvis. Its cell salt is Silicea, or Silica, (Cell Salt #12), which is recommended for addressing brittle bones, as well as to strengthen emotional and mental grit. It is known for healing skin, connective tissues, hair, and nails.

CAPRICORN

Capricorn is the ruler of bones, joints, knees, and teeth. Capricorn's nature is dependable and serious, but also rigid and inflexible at times. Capricorns resist change and can be stubborn, unforgiving, and hard on themselves and others. Calcarea Phosphorica (Cell Salt #2) is Capricorn's birth salt, and it is appropriately also the cell salt for bone strength, calcium absorption, and injury recovery.

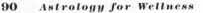

AQUARIUS

Aquarians are forward-thinking, open-minded intellectuals who love free-flowing ideas. Aquarius' cell salt is Natrum Muriaticum (Cell Salt #9), which helps regulate water in the body's cells and tissues whenever there is an imbalance of moisture in the body. Other body areas governed by Aquarius are the circulatory system, lower legs, ankles, and also the wrists.

PISCES

Pisceans are artistic, dreamy, and sensitive. They like to help others and tend to sacrifice for those they love. Pisces rules the immune system and the feet. Their birth salt is Ferrum Phosphoricum (Cell Salt #4) which carries oxygen to every cell in the body and helps speed recovery in the early stages of a fever, inflammation, and colds. It supports the action of all other cell salts.

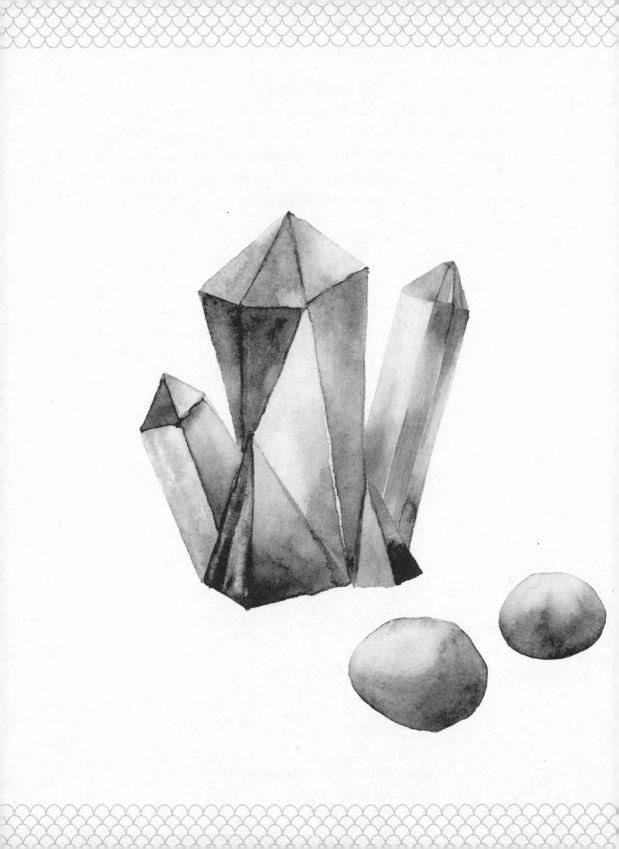

6

Healing Crystals

&

Power Stones

Crystals can help serve as spiritual power tools to teach us how to bring the mind to a greater sense of peace, the body into a more stable, grounded state, and the spirit into connection with the infinite from which springs all creation. Gemstones can remind us of a higher truth and keep us centered in that light.

When we become aware of the qualities of beauty, frequency, and color and their possible uses, stone "medicine" may help us explore what our current needs are and how we may transform certain situations by using a stone as a meditative focus and an inspirational power source. Gems and minerals have patterns and pictures on their surfaces that can transport us to another world, igniting our imagination. They are very tactile and soothing to touch and hold.

The idea of healing with crystals was first popularized in the 1930s when the famous American trance psychic Edgar Cayce claimed that his visions revealed that in the time of Atlantis crystals were used as a source of energy. He even described a crystal capstone on a centrally located pyramid that could power airships. He also mentioned specific stones when prescribing healing protocols for the people he read for.

According to crystal researcher Marcel Vogel, a senior scientist with IBM for twenty-seven years, "The crystal is a neutral object whose inner structure exhibits a state of perfection and balance. . . . Like a laser, it radiates energy in a coherent, highly concentrated form, and this energy may be transmitted into objects or people at will. With proper training, a healer using a crystal can release negative thought forms which have taken shape as disease patterns."

A gemstone or even just a stone becomes a meditative amplifier that can help to transform situations. Stones can keep us centered and reminded of a higher truth. By looking to the mineral kingdom for assistance in the healing process, we are connecting to tools that enable us to look deeper within in order to obtain an understanding of the cause of the distress that is creating disease. Distress can be caused by negative beliefs, by environmental factors, or by interactions with other people, which can sometimes create havoc in our energy field. When we consume alcohol or drugs, we can also affect our energy fields and cause a disruption in our vibrations.

Always remember that crystal healing should be used in conjunction with—and not as a substitute for—conventional medicine. There are many factors that contribute to well-being. Illnesses need to be tended to by a trusted physician. However, stress and distress can also have a profound effect on heath. All thoughts and actions have consequences, creating harmony or disharmony. Disharmony can cause illness. Working with ritual and with healing rocks and crystals can help you to create harmony, handle your stress, and feel better.

Your healing stones offer a beautiful stability and can help you focus on your strengths so that you can use them to compensate for your weaknesses. When we use crystals or stones as healing tools, they have the ability to rebalance a disruptive vibration so that we can be aware of the reason behind the distress.

Below we describe the nature and special healing message of crystals for each sign of the zodiac. We have gathered the information for these astrological associations through working with them for many years, and we suggest the perfect power stone for each sign.

ARIES: GARNET

The garnet takes its name from the resemblance of its deep red color to that of the pomegranate. It can help bring success in things you passionately believe in and, if appropriate, can flame the sparks of sexual energy. It may also be useful when wisdom and balance are needed in this most important exchange of energies. If this is so, look within to see if true love, tenderness, and genuine respect and caring are part of your romantic passion.

Garnet can help bring balance and self-awareness and destroy flightiness, leaving in its place love, romance, and sometimes lustiness, for those who need it.

Because of its rich color and association with the root chakra, the garnet suggests a powerful influence for sensuality and sexuality. It may help put you in touch with your animal instincts, enabling you to act and react with pure body wisdom. Therapists who recognize the power of gemstones use the garnet in counseling couples whose sexual chemistry has begun to wane.

For meditation and ritual purposes, the garnet is used primarily as a power stone to enhance self-confidence and to help manifest personal and career goals. Garnet has properties useful for giving inspiration during times of confusion. The red garnet is a stone of profound love and helps to ensure fidelity in relationships. It is a stone of patience and persistence and is also emblematic of spiritual awareness and compassion.

Garnet is highly versatile—it encourages the wearer to search for answers—and the answers that come as a result of this search will be helpful and important ones. Worn on a regular basis, the stone is believed to boost energy and stimulate romantic love.

Garnet's message: Because it has a bold energy, the garnet makes a perfect amulet for someone whose confidence or self-esteem needs bolstering. Because of its warm vibrations, it makes a good meditation stone for security and intimacy.

Other good gemstones for Aries are bloodstone, red jasper, and pyrite.

TAURUS: ROSE QUARTZ

Rose quartz is the stone that can help heal the heart, because it works on an emotional level. It can help you to become more aware of the love that is all around you and can assist you in getting in touch with your emotions. Rose quartz teaches us to love ourselves more, thus opening us up to a greater universal love. When we don't love ourselves fully, we are wounded inside, and a

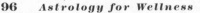

wound will always cry out to be healed. Rose quartz heals emotional wounds by giving compassion and comfort. It can be used to help overcome grief.

Rose quartz's properties include inner peace, tranquility, and all matters dealing with giving and receiving affection.

Unlike the hard-edged, pointed crystals of clear quartz, the lovely rose quartz is found in great veins running through Mother Earth like her life's blood. Use it when compassion and generosity need to be shown or when healing and forgiveness are needed. Rose quartz may help those who have suffered through trauma and the pain of an unhappy childhood. If this is true for you, start by forgiving yourself and others. Be gentle with yourself and others; we have all suffered wounds. From forgiveness can come a path to true healing.

You can also sleep with rose quartz next to you on a bedside table. The pain of a difficult past problem may come up in dreams, but you can better handle it if you affirm before you go to sleep that you are ready to forgive yourself and others and to release all pain from past events.

Rose quartz's message: Self-fulfillment and inner peace require you to love and nurture yourself and those you care about. Work on how to give love as well as how to receive it. Remember to forgive.

Other good gemstones for Taurus are emerald, malachite, and selenite.

GEMINI: AGATE

Agate is a general protector of the entire body and the entire auric field. Agate can help us to focus on growth and healing. It attracts strength and vitality, and it has the ability to help bring the body into balance. A special property of agate is the blending and balancing of energies for power, protection, and organizational qualities, causing a stabilizing effect. Agate also can help reinforce the body's connection to the earth. It can give courage and dispel fears, all of which increase self-confidence. It gives us the strength to carry on, even when we feel weak or tired.

Agate offers protection from bad dreams. It also protects us from stress and worry. Agates with banded colors placed at the head of a sleeper are said to give rich and varied dreams.

Since our earliest civilizations, agates have been prized gems. They were used in jewelry and as spiritual power tools in Babylonia. Conjurers in Persia used the crystal to try to affect the weather. In ancient Asia, agates were used to see the future. Studying the circular patterns helped open the pathway to receive guidance and messages by connecting the pathways between the conscious and subconscious minds.

Agate can also be enlisted for emotional healing, especially to resolve bitterness and resentments. It is believed to be a stone of harmony and, therefore, can help soften feelings of envy by dissipating agitation. By bringing the elements of one's being into harmony, it can improve how one functions in relationships. Agate also enhances creativity and stimulates the intellect. Carry a pocket-size piece of agate when you have to make an important decision.

Agate's message: Placing an agate on a bedside table may aid with insomnia and can stimulate pleasant dreams. If you have to deal with numbers, an agate placed on your desk will help you be more precise. You'll also be more analytical as well as creative in your approach to situations.

Other good gemstones for Gemini are clear quartz, tiger's eye, and bi-colored tourmaline.

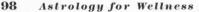

CANCER: CARNELIAN

Carnelian grounds energy and helps us to pay attention to the present moment, thus teaching us to focus and manifest our personal power. Use it to encourage strength and the courage to prevail. Carnelian helps to ease stress and anxiety and to improve memory.

Use carnelian when barriers of time and space or discouraging news threaten to stop you on your path. If this is true for you now, it is necessary for you to look below the surface of things in order for you to know what is really going on, for things are usually not what they seem. There is no reason to give up unless and until you know exactly how things stand. Once you know, carnelian can help you regain your courage.

Carry carnelian with you to guard against those who try to use their power over you. It can also help you regain the drive you need to pursue your goals or help to give birth to a new project or flesh out an existing one. Believed to prevent depression, carnelian helps to build courage by providing self-esteem and an optimistic outlook.

Carnelian stimulates energy, physical power, and courage and helps to ground you on the physical plane.

Early Egyptians used carnelian for amulets, as it was thought to protect the wearer from evil and to prevent anger and envy. Renaissance mystics kept carnelian amulets in their homes as protection against curses.

Carnelian's message: It offers patience while counteracting doubt and negative thoughts. It also assists in decision-making by helping us ground ourselves in the present and make decisions based not on our past but on our present reality.

Other good gemstones for Cancer are kunzite, ammonite, and moonstone.

LEO: CITRINE

The citrine's sunny color helps restore the mind in much the same way that basking in the life-giving light of the Sun does. Citrine helps us maintain a positive outlook on life. It removes blocks and fears on all levels and helps us to better communicate with others. Citrine helps create a sense of stability, adds energy and emotional balance, and provides a rational approach to things, grounding us in the here and now.

Citrine's energy means that a positive, optimistic attitude will produce a positive outcome. Use it when great self-confidence and self-esteem are needed. Stress and fatigue, either emotional or physical, can make life seem bleak and can make you unable to cope with challenges. Make sure to get enough rest and have some fun. Citrine can help you regain your emotional balance. We all stray from our path. How long it takes us to recover is what determines our successes and failures.

Citrine is one of the best stones for manifesting power on both a practical and a magical level. Because it encourages a healthy ego, self-esteem, and feelings of worth, it empowers its wearer both emotionally and spiritually. Many healers who use crystals in their practice believe that the stone can increase the significance of dreams and open the mind to new and more positive thought forms. Due to its color, it is believed to strengthen the urinary and endocrine systems.

Citrine is known to clean toxic impurities in the air and aura. On the metaphyscial level, it is thought to boost willpower, happiness, and confidence while reducing self-destructive tendencies. As a result, it can also bring good fortune, often in surprising ways.

Citrine's message: Some therapists believe that people who are have lost a sense of their individual identity because of an unhappy or abusive

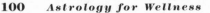

relationship can reclaim much of their personal power by regularly meditating with citrine.

Other good gemstones for Leo are amber, topaz, and jasper.

VIRGO: JADE

This stone acts in a protective way, on both the physical and spiritual levels. Jade has long been believed to facilitate and fortify a long and peaceful life. The Chinese have traditionally held jade in very high esteem, and it has a lovely history as a protective talisman that can alleviate the worry and anxiety that Virgo is prone to.

Amulets of animals were carved from jade to promote a healthier life and attract spiritual protection when needed. Jade was also used in rituals to attract wealth and fortune. Jade statues for abundance and protection were common. Dishes were often carved from jade. The gem was also believed to facilitate longevity, and therefore, food or drink in jade vessels would absorb that energy.

Jade energy bestows peace, calmness, harmony, tranquility, and mental clarity and encourages the safe expression of true feelings and emotions. It strongly influences matters of the heart and can help to improve relationships. Jade is wonderful for repairing relationship connections and ties that have been lost or broken.

Jade inspires and promotes creative thought. This stone also promotes a more unified environment so you may use it to develop the ability to compromise with partners, family members, or coworkers.

In business matters, you can use jade to unite individuals with differing—and sometimes conflicting—agendas and get them working toward common goals. It aids in creating a harmonious atmosphere and a desire for success and abundance without materialism or greed.

Jade is also favored for strengthening clear reasoning and, in so doing, stimulating excellent decision-making. Because it has a balancing effect, jade motivates wearers to believe that their plans and ambitions are worthy of success.

Jade's message: This is a helpful stone for those who have a nervous temperament or who are easily overwhelmed. The loving energies of this stone will assist you in recovering from emotional trauma because it provides grounding energy and a sense of security.

Other good gemstones for Virgo are amazonite, sapphire, and zircon.

LIBRA: TURQUOISE

One of the most ancient protection stones, turquoise has long been used in sacred rituals associated with sky energy because of its color and because it also brings sky energy down to earth. Prized in Asian as well as Native American cultures, it is known as a multipurpose stone, excellent for promoting a sense of self-awareness and the ability to communicate honestly and from the heart. The stone encourages creative thinking—as many do—but turquoise has the power to help channel that creative energy in a productive and useful way that benefits the user and the community as a whole.

Turquoise is considered a lucky stone; it facilitates the attraction of abundance and prosperity. Turquoise has a balancing influence that assists decision-making. Its properties include inducing mental relaxation, stress reduction, confidence, attunement, and physical well-being.

The blue-green turquoise is a stone sacred to many cultures around the world. Use it when you feel the need to call on your spirit guides because you have reached an important time in your life or you are at a crossroads. Turquoise is helpful when you need to restore communication with your

Higher Self, and it stimulates your development on the spiritual level. If this is true for you now, it is time to take action to restore your faith. Life often appears meaningless when our faith in the unseen forces that surround and sustain us is weak.

Turquoise can help us not to be distracted by our sorrows. It can help restore our sense of humor so we can enjoy life's gifts as well as its challenges, for we cannot have one without the other. Miracles can be seen every day. Turquoise is a favorite stone among metaphysical healers, who believe that it has the power to energize the body and spirit as well as to balance right brain–left brain disparity.

Turquoise's message: True communication is about more than words, and turquoise can help achieve this. Carrying a piece of turquoise will help keep you centered, and wearing it improves all the senses, including the sixth sense.

Other good gemstones for Libra are diamond, blue topaz, and lepidolite.

SCORPIO: OBSIDIAN

Obsidian is a stone of protection that prevents you from becoming emotionally drained by others. It can work as a shield against unwanted vibrations and help protect you from physical or emotional harm. Native Americans keep this stone on them as protection against negative energies or psychic attack.

Obsidian tends to give emotional stability in times of high stress, in part by preventing energy from draining out of the body. The energy to help with grounding is the strongest attribute of this stone. Keeping obsidian with you helps prevent negative thought patterns and can also be used for space clearing because it is known to remove vibrations of unhelpful or distracting entities.

Obsidian is an excellent crystal-gazing tool. Some practitioners have better success peering into obsidian's black depths to reach their subconscious messages than into a traditional clear quartz crystal ball.

The black glasslike obsidian is forged in the fires of volcanoes, Mother Earth's way of clearing away the old to make way for the new. It helps with transitions, so use it when you realize that the old must be completely released before the new can enter your life. It may also be useful when obsessions and negative thoughts and actions are blocking you. If this is happening to you, try to let every negative thought and action you encounter in yourself or in others remind you to think and act positively.

This gemstone may help you recover forgotten abilities within yourself. Obsidian can help you to become more aware of your true place in the universe by sharpening your inner vision. It will also help you become more aware of your imperfections and at the same time provide constructive solutions and insights.

Obsidian's message: Do not give in to the desire to think and act negatively even if others do. This is a difficult but most-powerful teaching. Our negativity comes back in unpleasant ways. Obsidian may help you cope with negativity and keep you centered in unstable times. Do not resist change.

Other good gemstones for Scorpio are onyx, ruby, and black opal.

SAGITTARIUS: AMETHYST

The amethyst's purple color, the color of pure spirit and the seemingly magical things connected with it, is rare in nature. Use it when you need approval from the universe or when peace and calm are needed. If this is so, try this basic meditation: Take a few moments to breathe calmly and focus your attention on your breathing. Let all thoughts drift away like clouds. After a while you may sense the small voice of your Higher Self. Be aware of the natural fear of not being in control or not knowing exactly what to do next on your path. Amethyst can help you trust yourself and "let go and let God/Goddess." Holding an amethyst may help ease the pain and sorrow of a loss or defeat.

Easily recognizable for its beautiful color, this stone is known to promote personal serenity and feelings of peace. Amethyst derives its reputation as a healing stone from ancient and medieval times when it was used as an amulet against drunkenness. The amethyst is a power stone on many levels and holds the intention to heal the body as well as the spirit. The amethyst has long been used to open people's psychic centers.

In folklore, this stone is believed to have a soothing and relaxing effect. Holistic healers sometimes use amethyst to ease toothache and bruising. It calms an overactive mind and brings a sense of tranquility to those who are frazzled by overwork. It is used as a dream stone and to help insomnia. For those who are psychically sensitive, it can improve the ability of second sight. As an amulet, it can be a talisman, worn to protect against jealousy, envy, and deception.

Amethyst's message: Amethyst is believed to be helpful in the treatment of insomnia. By putting an amethyst under the pillow, a troubled sleeper should experience better REM sleep, with less chance of fitful slumber.

Other good gemstones for Sagittarius are sodalite, sugilite, and tanzanite.

CAPRICORN: AMBER

Amber is the oldest geological specimen to be used in jewelry. Archeologists digging primitive sites near the Baltic Sea have found evidence of amber jewelry that is approximately forty thousand years old.

This good-luck stone brings together the purifying, revitalizing force of the Sun and the absorptive, transmuting energy of the planet we walk on to create a powerful metaphysical tool. In mythology, Apollo cried amber tears after being banished from Olympus. Medieval housewives would burn amber to bring good energy into their homes. Native American tribal healers used it in fire ceremonies.

Ancient Greeks discovered that if they rubbed a piece of amber vigorously, it became electrically charged. The early name for amber was *electron*, which is the root word for today's *electricity*. Amber's use as a treasured spiritual power tool reaches back to humans' earliest history.

Amber absorbs negative energy, helps to ground one to the earth plane, and protects the sensitive person. It helps to distribute vitality to our aura, and it centers people during meditation. Amber can be worn or carried to help calm the nerves. Amber allows people to receive from the universe, yet assists them to remain physically alert.

Amber is not technically a crystal but is an organic compound. Some 360 million years ago, extinct pine trees oozed thick, sticky resins. As these resins flowed, a variety of living and decomposing matter became trapped inside. Then the resin fossilized under the great pressure from the earth's changes. Many ancient traditions associate amber with the universal life force because, essentially, actual life has been trapped inside.

Amber's message: Amber is excellent at removing self-imposed obstacles to any projects. It enhances a constructive way of behaving, fueled by self-confidence. It can attract new friendships and aid in focusing your intentions for manifestation, helping you to reach your goals.

Other good gemstones for Capricorn are jet, smoky quartz, and chrysoprase.

AQUARIUS: LAPIS LAZULI

Mother Nature seems to have used the deep blue lapis lazuli to capture the sky in solid form. The glittering pyrite inclusions against the deep blue backdrop of this splendid stone create a striking likeness of a galaxy. Lapis is an excellent stone to help with peaceful sleep and psychic dreaming. It can bring matters more clearly to the mind. The stone will allow for cosmic communication with other dimensions of reality. Sleeping with this gemstone on a night table next to your bed can help you see the meaning in your dreams more clearly by allowing you to interpret and understand the messages or information that your subconscious is providing.

Use lapis to help with success in business and other worldly pursuits that benefit large portions of humanity. It is good to use for humanitarian quests and interests as it has far-reaching effects. Early cultures valued lapis more than gold. In Egypt it was customary to bury a lapis scarab with the dead, as it was believed to offer protection. It is also believed to enhance higher love, powers of intelligence, and concentrated intention.

Lapis can help you focus on the cooperation of universal brotherhood and sisterhood to produce abundance. Some other properties of lapis are illumination, wisdom, mental insight, and clarity of thought. It may also help when systems of information exchange, transportation, and communication are blocked. Lapis can help you to communicate your deeply felt beliefs and put them into practice in the outer world. It can help shy, introverted people express themselves. Expressing your true self can free energies you would otherwise waste repressing. Lapis helps to release old, buried emotions, thereby helping to dispel depression.

Lapis lazuli's message: Meditate with lapis when you need all methods of moving people, services, and facts to be as direct and simple as possible. Use it when you need a higher perspective on your situation. When blocked channels are cleared by lapis, expect energies to be a bit chaotic initially, before they calm down.

Other good gemstones for Aquarius are fluorite, azurite, and labradorite.

PISCES: OPAL

The opal owes its fiery beauty to the refractions of tiny imperfections and water trapped within its crystalline cells. The dance of color in opal is the result of light being radiated by microscopic silica spheres. Watching the colors flash when luminous sparkles flicker within an opal gemstone leaves you with little doubt that this is a beautiful and powerful crystal.

An opal may bring you enlightenment, integrity, or even the fires of romance. It enhances the emotions and amplifies personal traits. Opal can assist you with almost any aspect of your life, such as joy, love, or success. Let your opal fire up your heart's desire and make your wishes come true. Opal helps magnetize opportunities for things to happen in exciting new ways. Use opal to call in good luck and good fortune, to initiate prosperity consciousness, and to encourage new ideas.

Opal acts as a magnet by helping to illuminate your interests and ability to see great possibilities. It encourages you to dance your life by amplifying your emotions and heightening your experiences.

There are two main opal categories, common and precious. Precious opals are those with the famous rainbow sparkles. Common opals are stones without fire.

If you are bored or in a rut, either type of opal can spark a flame of passion and ignite your imagination, helping you see solutions to mundane problems. It turns up the power in everything.

Adding this gemstone to any prayer, ritual, or creative work will strengthen your intention and affirmation. Shamans use opals in important ceremonies such as vision quests. For divination and oracle use, you may want to wear or hold an opal. It will enhance your attunement to the messages of the tarot or other divination readings.

Opal's message: It magnifies your thoughts and feelings and promotes all intuitive abilities. In ancient times the opal was thought to be a very powerful healing stone and was believed to open up the senses of the third eye. The opal can be a doorway to your spiritual awareness.

Other good gemstones for Pisces are aquamarine, coral, and pearl.

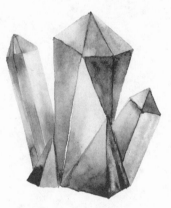

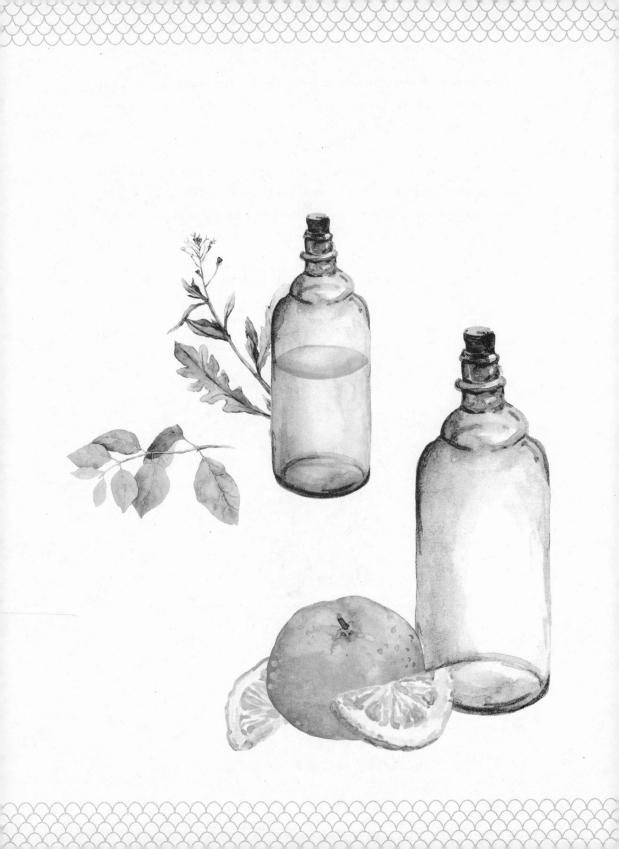

7

Astrology, Aromatherapy & Sign Scents

Creating your own aromatherapy is a lovely way to make magic. The right mixes of essential oils and other botanical and mineral-based ingredients can produce optimum benefits for your body, mind, and spirit.

You will also find the aroma-therapeutic effects of the following easy-to-find oils and scents to be restorative and revitalizing. Just add a few drops to your bath, infuse a cotton ball with the essential oil, and inhale the aroma, or add to water in a spray bottle and spritz the air when you feel you need an extra-special boost to soothe and uplift your personal space.

◇◇◇◇◇◇◇◇◇◇◇◇◇◇◇◇◇◇◇◇◇◇◇◇◇◇◇◇◇◇◇◇

» Choose 100 percent pure, organic essential oil

» Fill an empty and unused mist-spray bottle with 4 fluid ounces (or 120 ml) of purified water.

» Add 20 drops of the oil to the water.

» Once you've added your essential oils to the water in the small spray bottle, screw the cap back on snugly, shake it gently to mix the ingredients

» We energize the finished mixture with our intention, seeing in our mind's eye the successful future result of its desired use.

» Use as needed. Usually two or three spritzes are sufficient for what you'll be using it for, but it's okay to use more.

» After use, store the mist bottle in a cool, dark place to protect the contents.

◇◇◇◇◇◇◇◇◇◇◇◇◇◇◇◇◇◇◇◇◇◇◇◇◇◇◇◇◇◇◇◇

ARIES

Arians are honest, brave, and headstrong. Their fiery, assertive, and coura-geous natures are full of charm and charisma. They favor stimulating and bold scents, rich and spicy ones that pervade their space with comfort and glowing warmth.

Frankincense and rosemary can help support the strong Aries energy, and peppermint can help cool and calm as well as help heal headaches, which Aries are prone to. Fragrant notes with hints of warming ginger, pepper, and clove are snappy penetrating scents that stimulate, purify, and invigorate, to complement the wild-child Aries who loves to unleash the free spirit within.

TAURUS

The best kind of scent for a kind, earthy, patient, practical Taurus is a luxu-rious blend of rich, sweet, creamy flowers such as honeysuckle, gardenia, or magnolia, to encourage feelings of protection and security. Taurus types are loyal, pragmatic, and good-humored.

Taurus relishes harmony. Beautiful art and music and delicious smells are important to a Taurus, as this sign is ruled by Venus, the planet of love and affection. To nurture their sensual nature try patchouli and ylang-ylang. Hyssop and wild cherry will help alleviate the sore throats that sometimes bother Taurus types.

GEMINI

Geminis are witty, changeable, versatile, talkative, well read. Inside of all Geminis there are actually two different people with two different sets of tastes. Those born under this sign love to communicate and put their point across. They know how to keep everyone interested. Basil, bergamot and grapefruit are great to inhale for nurturing an overactive mind.

Their need for mental stimulation might also suggest a light hint of mint or citrus and multitasking with lavender and lily of the valley to create an inspiring, joyful, and positive environment and improve concentration. Eucalyptus can help with respiratory problems, if needed.

CANCER

Cancerians are caring, tenacious, and sensitive. Those born under the astrological sign Cancer are well known for their ability to nurture and protect others. Feelings and the moods they produce are an important part of being a Cancerian.

To stay comforted and centered, they might be drawn to the protective aromas of melon, vanilla, and coconut. Other good oils are sandalwood and lavender to help stimulate a sense of peace and emotional well-being, which in turn, facilitates the release of repressed negative emotions, allowing them to be addressed and then released.

Chamomile and mint are good for aiding digestion.

LEO

Loving Leo rules the creative process. Leos are dramatic, proud, organized, romantic, playful, and fun. Leos need to be complimented and admired. They demand attention. They can show the world how to really live and laugh and love the good life. Lemon and ginger oils help sore backs, sometimes a tender area for Leo, and garlic and marjoram are good for the heart.

A lovely royal scent would be something with cinnamon, mandarin, and nutmeg to stimulate creativity, desire, focus, and motivation; help support a positive attitude; and magnify a Leo's life purpose.

VIRGO

Virgo is an earth sign. People born during this time are energetic, analytical, intelligent, reliable, and responsible. They have their feet on the ground and possess the gift of discernment. They like scents that are clean and simple, yet special. Virgos are often meticulous perfectionists.

To alleviate some of their worries, they can benefit from patchouli, Melissa, and chamomile, which will help to calm the nervous system, soothing feelings of being overwhelmed with an overworked mercurial mind. Rain, cedar, or grass would also refresh and remind a Virgo to be grounded and close to nature.

LIBRA

Faithfulness, partnership, and loyalty are essential to a Libra. They want to be surrounded by the best. Libra is an air sign, and ideas and happy thoughts are important to them. Cedar inspires steadiness for the sometimes indecisive Libra.

For their refined tastes and keen perceptiveness, we suggest loving and peaceful neroli (orange blossom) and lavender to help achieve balance and harmony and to enhance their appreciation of beauty. Rose is relaxing, soothing, and helps to strengthen the Libran's inner being—gentle but strong, it has an uplifting effect on the psyche and a balancing effect.

SCORPIO

Scorpios are intense, loyal, and determined. They are the master detectives of the zodiac. Scorpios like to discover the hidden truth. They have strong passions, so strong aromas appeal.

Jasmine nurtures their sensual side, and geranium can help soften their intense nature.

Scorpios are the embodiment of Oscar Wilde's brilliant statement, "I can resist anything except temptation." The enticing scents of wisteria, anise, or tuberose will suit their sexy natures and help them appreciate their mystical powers. It also will help to heal past traumas to the energy field and boundary violations.

SAGITTARIUS

Those born under the sign of Sagittarius are optimistic and enthusiastic and have a love of travel, animals, the great outdoors, natural healing, and all things foreign and exotic. You can expect them to be surprisingly blunt and honest about their likes and dislikes.

Jupiter, the planet of good fortune, rules them. Tea tree is an essential oil that will help heal and encourage a Sagittarian spirit. Jasmine, saffron, or cinnamon would transport the adventurous traveler within to the exotic locales they are drawn to, along with relieving the tensions of travel.

CAPRICORN

Capricorns are ambitious, prudent, and self-disciplined. They have very deep and real emotional needs that can slow them down, but their persistence and ability to focus on a goal enables them to succeed. Coriander is suitable for softening their hard-headed and stubborn side.

Capricorns can also be surprisingly sensuous. Vetiver or sage with a hint of musk would suit this earthy sign, a personality that appreciates tradition, meaning, and loyalty. Pine promotes feelings of strength, empowerment, and protection that are a result of being close to nature.

AQUARIUS

Aquarians are unique, brilliant, articulate, and progressive. They have free-thinking minds, unfettered by rules. They like inventing, experimenting, and discovering. Aquarians thrive on being rebellious and different. They are futuristic but also students of history, so they will appreciate a scent that harkens back to another time. Cypress is a good choice.

To help de-stress this idealistic intellectual, try the delightful scent of lemon verbena with amber or almond to foster feelings of determination to leave the past behind so that they can move forward.

PISCES

Pisces are very sensitive, full of inspiration and clairvoyance. They can experience scents on a deeply mystical soul level, feeling the subtle energies of the various ingredients. Elemi is a perfect stress reducer and meditation oil for a Pisces.

A Piscean's natural ability to be empathetically connected requires an aroma such as ylang-ylang to protect them from negativity, to reduce self-consciousness, and to complement their dreamy, spiritual nature. Lilac is also good and peach or mango would appeal because of the sweet aroma of their oils.

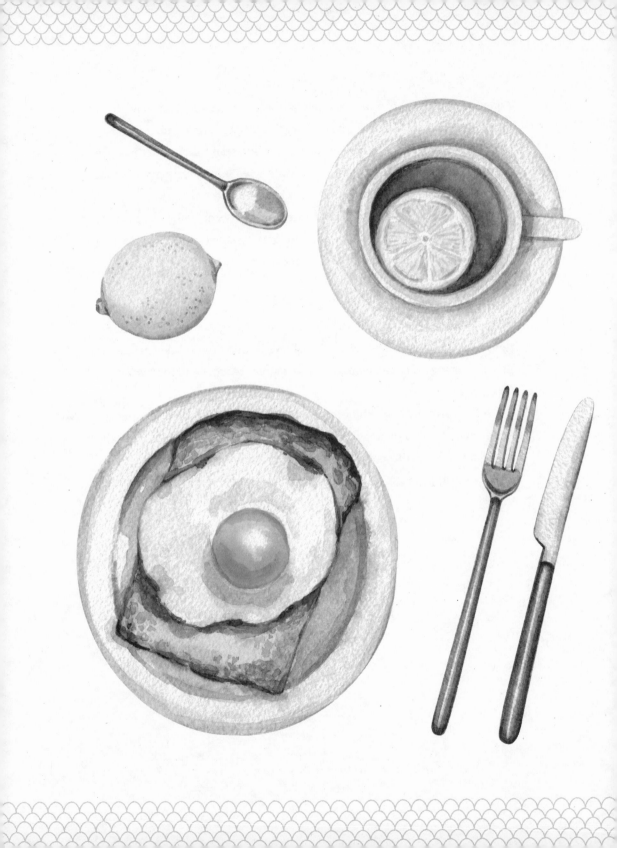

8

Breakfast Foods & Snacks

Eating the right breakfast or snack for your astro personality can make the difference between having an amazing day and one that's less than ideal. Here are suggestions of foods that might make you start the day on the best note, or refuel you as a snack, based on your zodiac sign.

ARIES

Knowing an Aries is like having your own military general on call, always ready, willing, and able to help you plan your campaign. For some morning or afternoon fuel and fun for an energy-burning fire sign, try carrot cupcakes topped with cream-cheese-and-maple-syrup frosting, packed with walnuts, honey, carrots, eggs, and almond flour to feed the inner child of a Ram on the run.

Aries usually favors anything that can be made quickly.

Arians also like brash, exciting flavors with bright notes of lemon, herbs, garlic, and olive oil that are served in small bites. Arians burn up energy fast. Try adding protein-packed red adzuki beans to salads and soups to stay fueled. Sometimes Arians need a fourth or even fifth meal!

For someone who's raring to go, forward flavors and foods with fiery, piquant, bold tastes are what Arians crave; sweets aren't nearly as appealing as salty snacks with a hit of cayenne, and they prefer cooling beverages with intense flavors like ginger.

TAURUS

Taureans value a middle-of-the-road approach to life. Not likely to get caught up in the latest trend, they believe in being themselves and often have a big appetite for all things delicious. The phrase "haste makes waste" expresses Taurus' viewpoint in a nutshell. Taureans love creamy classics that they can savor, so a piece of cheesy cheddar quiche or a velvety smoothie is perfect to feed the hungry beast.

Taurus is all about the appreciation of living well, what can be touched and savored. They have a common-sense approach along with a fondness for the good life, luxury foods, and eating pleasure. That doesn't mean that they can't enjoy healthy foods, as long as the foods still taste delicious.

Taurus likes smoothies, so try adding a superpower like matcha, cacao, or green moringa powder.

If a food can pull off the feat of being rich and creamy yet still somehow nutritious (like avocado), it's got Taurus written all over it.

GEMINI

Geminis want to experience life fully and in as many different ways as they can. They have two opinions about everything, and sometimes they can't make up their minds, so a layered protein bar makes great morning snack, enabling them to eat on the run. Tahini or lemon bars with coconut flour, almond meal, spices, and rice malt syrup satisfy the variety that Gemini crave.

Their need for mental stimulation keeps them constantly on the go, and snacks and finger foods keep them energized. Gemini's mind is always working overtime, so a variety of brain foods such as turmeric, salmon, eggs, dandelion greens, and jícama should be added to the menu.

They tend to avoid foods that require them to sit and digest, preferring to eat and move on to the next interesting thing. Earthy foods such as mango, root vegetables, or feta cheese can also help keep Geminis grounded.

CANCER

More than those born under any other sign, Cancerians are driven by feelings and intuition. Even though they are intelligent, practical people, they use their feelings as a sort of radar, and a great many of their decisions are based on this radar. How about a nurturing, grounding start to the day in the form of warm fruit crisp, to add some sweet spice and comfort?

Drinking plenty of pure water and foods high in water content are good for them. They should never eat when they are upset because they occasionally transfer their emotional state to their digestive system and so may have a sensitive stomach.

Pickled and fermented foods such as kimchi, sauerkraut, and miso would be good for a Moon child's gut health. Comforting foods are the ones they love best; if something is homemade such as macaroni and cheese or rice pudding, they are sold.

LEO

The task can be big or small, complicated or relatively easy, but no matter what it is, Leo has a plan for how to get it done better, faster, more economically, and even with more style. She believes that her way is the only way, and will probably tell you so. A festive acai bowl with a dash of cinnamon, some orange juice, and some honey, makes a fast and colorful breakfast feast fit for a king or queen. Protein-rich seeds are good add-ons to morning cereal or yogurt snack—hemp, chia, or flax. Leos like rich!

Wise Leos will add what their doctor considers to be heart-healthy foods to the royal menu plan. The priciest fruits, the most expensive cheeses, the prize-winning chocolates—these are the snacks Leos gravitate toward. And there's a good chance a mini-meal will contain some kind of golden color.

VIRGO

Virgos are driven by the search for perfection in every way. The importance that Virgos place on perfection leads them to seek out the crème de la crème in all sorts of areas in life. Their craftiness, good taste, and pickiness are legendary. A frittata with basil, tomatoes, and mozzarella makes a pretty picture-perfect breakfast.

They can be picky eaters. Note that the wear and tear of responsibility can be often be exhausting to the Virgo perfectionist. Their meals are like a craft project to them; things are cut and diced precisely and plated to perfection.

As the sign that rules digestion, Virgo is especially keen on snacks with GI-friendly fiber and enzymes. Small amounts of aloe vera juice as well as prebiotics and probiotics will assist in helping maintain intestinal fortitude. And though thrifty, when it comes to buying groceries, they like food that's a little bit special.

LIBRA

Libras are driven by the desire to bring beauty and harmony to their world and the world at large. They have refined tastes and may actually recoil from things that are ugly, loud, or unpleasant. For many Libras, vulgarity is an affront. Libras would love the idea of adding edible flowers to garnish a dish, as they are all about beauty. Hibiscus, lavender, rose, and elderflower are ones to try.

They need a satisfying breakfast, with harmonious tastes and textures, something like an apple crumble with oats, cranberries, and sunflowers seeds, served with yogurt.

Libras do not like extremes and prefer dishes that are neither too spicy nor too bland. A Libran looks for a harmonious blend in all things. Eating is an art to them; they are the consummate epicures and their approach to culinary perfection requires that what they eat be absolutely fresh and also look picture perfect, even if it is just a 3:00 p.m. snack at their desk. A delicate soup, poached fruit straight from the farm, a plate of their favorite cheeses, or freshly baked bread—any of these could be satisfying to a Libra.

SCORPIO

Scorpios are keen students of psychology and always want to know what makes people do the things they do. Scorpios have a reputation for being emotional, mysterious, and secretive. Why not a breakfast cookie for those times when nothing else will do, after a particularly intense and passionate evening? A guilt-free chocolate chip cookie packed with healthy nutrients: oat flour, almond flour, cinnamon, eggs, and coconut palm sugar.

Their list of favorite foods will usually include some of those known to arouse passion, such as oysters, chocolate, asparagus, figs, or avocados, or those containing chiles. They get really into the sensuous, luxurious, sexy, satisfying experience of eating. They want their choices to weave a magic spell, and they crave intensity (so that's why those plain rice cakes never appealed). Foods that have pure, strong flavors and aromas are right up their alley. Maca can be added to foods—it is a powder from a plant with libido-boosting amino acids, zinc, and iron.

SAGITTARIUS

Sagittarians love to study and especially to teach. They can expand their understanding of the way the world works through travel, certainly, but also through travel in their mind via philosophy and learning. Breakfast tortillas with tomatoes, onions, garlic, and sweet and pungent peppers are typical of Mexican cooking and fuel up the Sagittarian urge for traveling through their day.

Sagittarians appreciate the best that other cultures and philosophies have to offer. Tasty foods with exotic traditions will spice up a Sagittarian's life—try harissa on eggs or tahini on naan bread.

They can be the most adventurous cooks and will attempt the most difficult recipes with hard-to-find ingredients. Lovers of nature, they are drawn to fresh foods that are minimally processed—something we all should be doing when those afternoon cravings strike. Their palate is wide ranging and, as people eager for new experiences, they will try almost anything.

CAPRICORN

Ask a Capricorn if you want a practical solution to a problem. The people born under this sign pride themselves on their common sense. They may not have a glamorous approach to problems, but they know how to get the job done. Potato pancakes with smoked salmon and dill crème fraîche are thin, crisp, and crunchy outside, a dependable and traditional dish, and a little indulgent—what Capricorns crave.

Capricorns like their meals to be regular and on time. Capricorns like to be respected for their choices and their knowledge about the food (and everything else). They know what they like and are not afraid to eat it every single day. No matter how their life changes, they have a strong allegiance to the foods with which they grew up. Earthy and traditional, like a hearty trail mix, would satisfy. Mushrooms and bone broth are also great ingredients for the grounded Capricorn.

AQUARIUS

The Aquarian mind is highly analytical and skilled at making quick assessments. Turning myriad information into easy-to-follow directions is never difficult for the people of this sign. Whipped polenta with parmesan, eggs, and sage makes a novel and filling breakfast—a bit of work to make but creates something different, which Aquarians love. Add sausage or bacon and it's a feast.

They are innovative and usually on the cutting edge of new thought regarding food as medicine. Freshness, sustainability, and humane farming are all are important to them. Aquarians are also interested in history and, therefore, would be open to trying some ancient grains including spelt, kamut, amaranth, and lupin in their snacks and baked goods.

Nonconformists like them have some pretty original ideas about food, which may explain the funny looks they have gotten while snacking on one of their vinegar-flavored experiments. When they eat alone at home, it's almost as if they are camping—no plates or utensils required.

PISCES

Pisces help you to understand that it is through compassion, caring, and a spirit that is open to receive the love of others that true happiness exists. Pisceans are plugged into the universe in a way that is otherworldly. They need to taste the sweetness of life. Poached pears in maple syrup, with apple juice, cloves, and raisins are easy and wholesome, a satisfying way to start the day.

Empathic more than any other sign, they need foods that restore balance, that lift the spirit, such as seafood, complex carbohydrates, seaweed, nuts, fruits, vegetables, rich with blues-beating nutrients. Many of them are vegetarians for moral reasons.

Delicate, gentle foods prepared simply are the ones that speak to them. And they may have a sweet tooth, too, thanks to their sweet-natured, dreamy outlook on life, and they long for sweetness in all areas. Pisces should always keep in mind that they have addictive personalities. Get creative with some "mocktail" recipes such as a watermelon-ginger spritzer or a grapefruit-basil mimosa to avoid the effects of alcohol but still get the sweetness Pisceans crave.

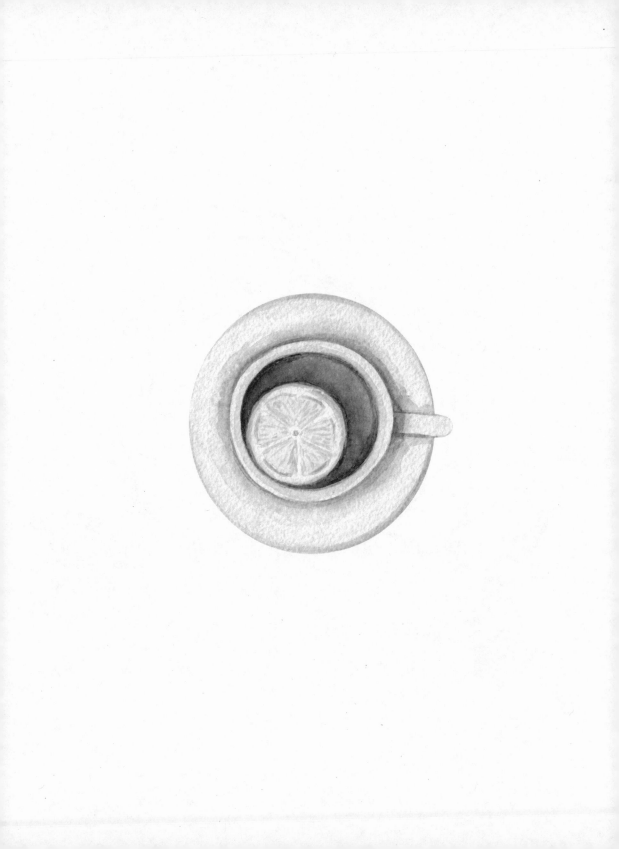

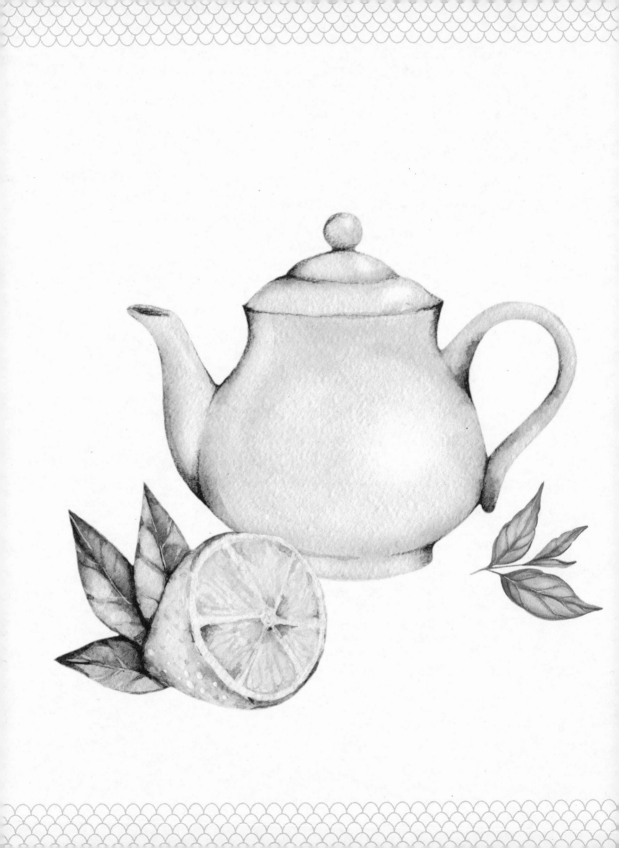

9

Nourishing Zodiac Tea Infusions

Herbal tea infusions are so good for you. An infusion is simply a strong tea made with one teaspoon dried herb for every cup of water. Infusions are great because they have medicinal properties and are hydrating (they count toward your daily water intake).

People are beginning to think of tea with the same reverence as coffee and recognize the range of its many varieties.

Teas are a wonderful way to contemplate the day, to plan your meals as you sip, and to take a few minutes to enjoy nourishing a healthy body, mind, and spirit.

When you perform a tea ritual regularly, and as you smell the infusions and drink, you start to think about your feelings and you naturally become more grateful and more intuitive.

Black, green, white, and oolong teas are all high in antioxidants, which make them all beneficial for general health and wellbeing.

TO PREPARE: Heat water until just boiling, pour it over the herb, cover the cup, let sit undisturbed 10–20 minutes. Try adding raw honey or fresh fruit juice before drinking.

ARIES: For an ambitious Aries, a spicy mix of black tea, cayenne, clove, and cardamom will fuel the desire to make things happen. They are so goal-oriented that they need a robust, assertive flavor that can kickstart a boost in energy and keep them going, as they always have a lot to do!

TAURUS: White tea infused with jasmine and peach creates a comforting, smooth brew that an industrious Taurus can relax with. Taurus like to plan for prosperity and growth while taking a time-out, sitting in a cozy chair with a delicious cup of tea to chase away stress.

GEMINI: A light blend of Assam with rose hips and allspice stimulates a Gemini's versatility and open mind. Geminis are a breath of fresh air, and their lively conversation over a cup of tea is always cheerfully entertaining. Iced or hot—you never know what this restless, quick-changer will crave!

CANCER: Cancerians love to nourish themselves and others. This pleasant, roasted mix is good as an after-dinner tea and will help soothe their sensitive stomachs. A blend of kuckicha, strawberry leaf, and angelica will help regulate emotions and give the nurturer a much-needed healing, reflective, restful break.

LEO: Earl Grey tea mixed with orange peel and lemongrass can enhance a Leo's confident, creative, charismatic personality. Leos love to entertain, and what's more fun than a tea party? This motivating, sunny brew will boost a drab day.

VIRGO: Peppermint and fenugreek tea will refresh and center a Virgo's mind. Virgos are always worrying about solving the problems in their daily life. Their morning cup of tea will sharpen their focus and calm their nerves, and even help them with sorting and organizing information.

LIBRA: A balanced union of white tea, red clover, and rose buds creates a lovely flavor. It will appeal to Libra's refined sense of harmony, as this is a meditative blend. Libras love to socialize over a cup of tea served in a beautiful teapot.

SCORPIO: A smoky blend of Lapsang Souchong tea, chocolate, and mango will help fuel a Scorpio's psychic energy. Sometimes they need a richly potent drink to transform their mood. Raspberry and lavender add sensual notes.

SAGITTARIUS: Sagittarians are always curious and exploring options. They love exotic spicy teas. A spirited combo of green tea with coconut and ginger flavors supplies Sagittarius with the passion and stamina they need for their next journey.

CAPRICORN: A black tea mixed with chicory and dandelion is the practical choice for giving the Goat a cup of of focused flavor. Capricorns work hard and need to retreat with a robust tea that they can depend on. Earthy flavors quiet the mind and nourish the bones.

AQUARIUS: For the idealistic trailblazer, flavorful licorice root, which promotes sustained energy release, will fuel Aquarius's visionary mind. Aquarians love to be inventive and hang with friends, often over a strong cup of tea. Sarsaparilla and ginseng teas will add excitement and focus and satisfy Aquarius's thirst for the unexpected.

PISCES: Sweet rooibos, white tea, and cinnamon flavors will support a Piscean's rich imagination. Pisceans love to get in touch with their creative and mystical nature by curling up in bed with a hot cup of tea. Chamomile and hibiscus are calming additions that help sooth a Piscean's sensitivity.

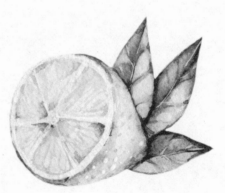

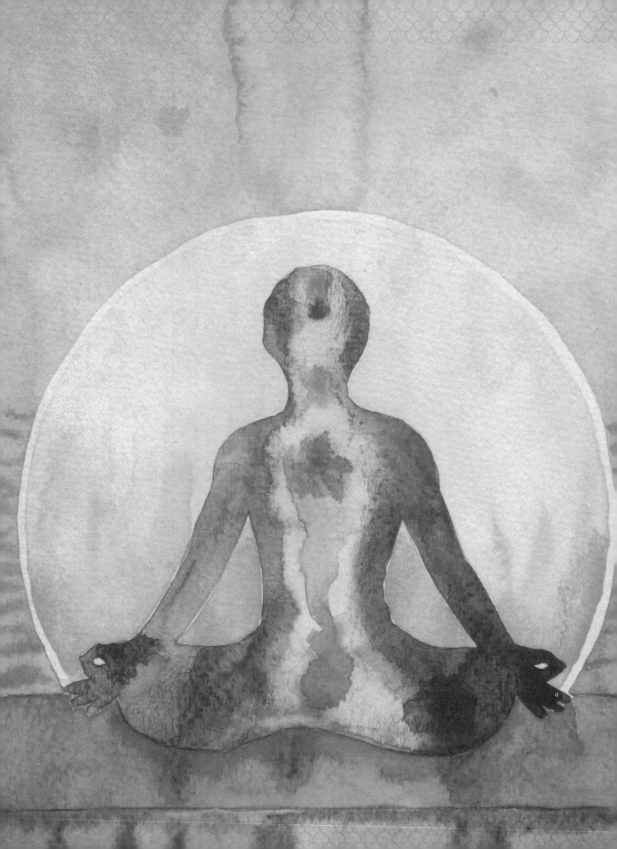

10

Yoga Poses

FOR EACH

Sign

In Sanskrit *yoga* means, "to unite." These poses (asanas) focus on the link between the traditional areas of the body in astrology and how we can strengthen them and unite our mind, body, and spirit through yoga. We are all subject to emotional upsets, anxiety, stress, depression, and anger at some point in life. Certain poses may be particularly helpful.

Note: You should always seek the advice of a physician or other qualified health-care provider before beginning any exercise program. If you experience any pain or difficulty with these exercises, stop and consult your health-care provider.

aries

Aries rules the head, brain, eyes, face, and muscles. Aries loves a challenge and has a will of steel. Aries may be prone to headaches. This pose builds stamina.

◇◇◇◇◇◇◇◇◇◇◇◇◇◇◇◇◇◇◇◇◇◇◇◇◇◇◇◇◇◇◇◇◇◇

WARRIOR POSE

» Stand tall with your feet 3 feet apart.

» Turn your right foot 90 degrees to the right and your left foot 30 degrees in the same direction.

» Pivot your pelvis to the right, turning it toward the front of your mat.

» Lift your arms to the sky. Bend your right knee so it is over your ankle.

» Hold for one minute.

» Repeat the pose, this time facing toward the left, reversing the directions above.

◇◇◇◇◇◇◇◇◇◇◇◇◇◇◇◇◇◇◇◇◇◇◇◇◇◇◇◇◇◇◇◇◇◇

taurus

Taurus rules the neck and throat, including the larynx, vocal cords, tonsils, thyroid, chin, lower jaw, ears, and tongue. This pose provides a steady, deliberate movement that nourishes a Taurus's patient personality.

◇◇◇◇◇◇◇◇◇◇◇◇◇◇◇◇◇◇◇◇◇◇◇◇◇◇◇◇◇◇◇◇◇◇◇

BOW POSE

» Lie on your stomach with your feet hip-width apart and your arms by the sides of your body.

» Bend your knees and hold your ankles.

» Breathing in, lift your chest off the ground and pull your legs up and back using your hands.

» Look straight ahead and smile!

» Stabilize the pose by paying attention to your breath. Once stabilized, your body is as taut as a bow.

» Continue to take long, deep breaths as you relax into Bow Pose. But don't get carried away! Be careful not to overdo the stretch.

» After 15–20 seconds, exhale and gently bring your legs and chest to the ground.

» Release your ankles and relax.

◇◇◇◇◇◇◇◇◇◇◇◇◇◇◇◇◇◇◇◇◇◇◇◇◇◇◇◇◇◇◇◇◇◇◇

gemini

Gemini rules the arms, hands, fingers, shoulders, upper ribs, lungs, and nervous system. These types are prone to nervousness, fidgeting, and "monkey mind" tendencies. Geminis are the communicators, so they tend to sit in front of a computer and can type for hours. They should be frequently rotating and relaxing their hands in between work. This pose is a good stretch for a Gemini.

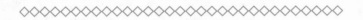

COBRA POSE

» Lie on your stomach with the top of your feet and chin resting on the floor. Keep your legs close together with your feet and heels lightly touching.

» Place your palms face down underneath your shoulders with your fingers pointing to the top of your mat. Keep your elbows parallel and hugged into your sides.

» Breathing in, gently lift your head, chest, and abdomen, while keeping your lower ribs, pelvis and navel pressed down on the mat.

» Draw your shoulders back and down away from your ears, opening your chest forward. Your gaze can be forward or to the sky, depending on the flexibility of your neck.

» Straightening your arms, slowly lift your chest off the floor while pressing down on the mat through your thighs. Make sure there is not too much weight in your palms. You can check by seeing if you can lift your hands off the mat to hover, while focusing on engaging your back muscles.

» Only straighten your arms to a point at which you feel a comfortable and natural. Hold the posture for up to 30 seconds.

» Breathing out to release, gently bring your abdomen, chest, and head back down to the floor.

◇◇

cancer

Cancer rules the breasts, breastbone, stomach, digestive system, lower ribs, womb, and pancreas. Forward folds will allow you to show yourself all the self-love, compassion, and protection you deserve. As you practice this pose, hold the intention of releasing emotions that do not serve your highest good and greatest joy.

◇◇

STANDING FORWARD BEND

» Start by standing and balancing your weight equally on both feet.

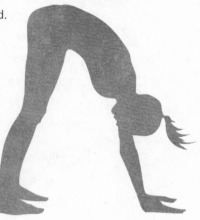

» Breathing in, extend your arms overhead.

» Breathing out, bend forward with a flat back and down toward your feet.

» Stay in the posture 20–30 seconds and continue to breath deeply.

» Keep your legs and spine erect with hands resting either on the floor, beside your feet, or on your legs.

» On an out breath, move your chest toward your knees and lift your hips and tailbone higher.

» Let your head relax and move it gently toward your feet. Keep breathing deeply.

» Breathing in, stretch your arms forward and up and slowly raise up to a standing position.

» Breathing out, bring your arms to the sides.

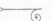

leo

Leo rules the heart, upper back, spine, spleen, and wrists. Leos have dynamic energy and love to play. This pose is helpful for back pain and opens the heart chakra.

◇◇◇◇◇◇◇◇◇◇◇◇◇◇◇◇◇◇◇◇◇◇◇◇◇◇◇◇◇◇◇◇◇

CAT STRETCH

» Place your hands and knees on the floor and your back in tabletop position.

» Your neck should be in a neutral position with your eyes gazing toward the floor.

» As you inhale, lift your chest and sit bones to the sky while also dropping your belly toward the floor; this should create a gentle arch in your back.

» Exhale and round your back toward the ceiling. Release your head between your arms so the crown of your head points toward the floor.

» Lift your head and look straight in front of you for several seconds.

» Inhale and move your spine back to neutral tabletop position, staying there for several seconds.

» Repeat the sequence 5 times.

◇◇◇◇◇◇◇◇◇◇◇◇◇◇◇◇◇◇◇◇◇◇◇◇◇◇◇◇◇◇◇◇◇

virgo

Virgo rules the sympathetic nervous system and lower digestive tract. Virgos thrive on organization and order. They are natural perfectionists and enjoy precision. This pose brings balance and equilibrium to the mind by embodying the graceful, steady stance of a tree.

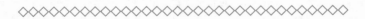

TREE POSE

» Stand tall and straight with arms by the sides of your body.

» Bend your right knee and place the right foot high up on your left thigh. The sole of the foot should be placed flat and firmly near the root of the thigh.

» Make sure that your left leg is straight. Find your balance.

» Once you are well balanced, take a deep breath in, gracefully raise your arms over your head from the side, and bring your palms together in Namaste *mudra* (hands-folded position).

» Look straight ahead in front of you at a distant object. A steady gaze helps maintain a steady balance.

» Ensure that your spine is straight. Your entire body should be taut, like a stretched elastic band. Keep taking in long, deep breaths. With each exhalation, relax the body more. Just be with the body and the breath with a gentle smile on your face.

» With slow exhalation, gently bring down your hands from the sides. You may gently release the right leg.

» Stand tall and straight as you did at the beginning of the posture. Repeat this pose with the left leg off the ground on the right thigh.

◇◇◇◇◇◇◇◇◇◇◇◇◇◇◇◇◇◇◇◇◇◇◇◇◇◇◇◇◇◇◇◇◇◇

libra

Libra rules the lumbar spine, kidneys, and adrenal glands. Librans are poised and elegant and they seek peace. This pose is a cross-legged posture that deepens the experience in meditation by calming the mind—connecting breaths with a balanced, open, and beautiful feeling.

◇◇◇◇◇◇◇◇◇◇◇◇◇◇◇◇◇◇◇◇◇◇◇◇◇◇◇◇◇◇◇◇◇◇◇

LOTUS POSE

» Sit on the floor or on a mat with legs stretched out in front of you, keeping your spine erect.

» Bend your right knee and place your foot on the left thigh. Make sure that the sole of your foot points upward and the heel is close to your abdomen.

» Repeat with your other leg.

» With both legs crossed and feet placed on opposite thighs, place your hands on your knees in mudra position.

» Keep your head straight and spine erect.

» Hold and continue with long, gentle breaths in and out.

» To come out of the pose, gently remove one foot at a time from your thighs.

◇◇◇◇◇◇◇◇◇◇◇◇◇◇◇◇◇◇◇◇◇◇◇◇◇◇◇◇◇◇◇◇◇◇◇

scorpio

Scorpio rules the genitals, bladder, and urinary tract. This pose stretches the inner thighs, improving flexibility in the groin and hip region, an amazing way to release stagnant emotions in the genital area. It also offers relief from menstrual discomfort and menopause symptoms

◇◇◇◇◇◇◇◇◇◇◇◇◇◇◇◇◇◇◇◇◇◇◇◇◇◇◇◇◇◇◇◇

BUTTERFLY POSE

» Sit with your spine erect and legs spread straight out.

» Bend your knees and bring your feet toward your pelvis. The soles of your feet should touch each other.

» Grab your feet tightly with your hands. You may place your hands underneath your feet for support.

» Make an effort to bring your heels as close to your groin as possible.

» Take a deep breath in. Breathing out, press your thighs and knees downward toward the floor. Make a gentle effort to keep pressing them downward.

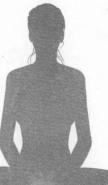

» Start flapping both your legs up and down like the wings of a butterfly. Start slow and gradually increase the speed. Continue to breathe normally.

»   Slow down and then stop. Take a deep breath in and
    as you exhale, bend forward, keeping your chin up and
    spine erect.

»   Press your elbows on your thighs or on your knees,
    pushing your knees and thighs closer to the floor.

»   Feel the stretch in your inner thighs and take long, deep
    breaths, relaxing the muscles more and more.

»   Take a deep breath in and bring your torso up.

»   As you exhale, gently release the posture. Straighten
    your legs out in front of you and relax.

◇◇◇◇◇◇◇◇◇◇◇◇◇◇◇◇◇◇◇◇◇◇◇◇◇◇◇◇◇◇◇

sagittarius

Sagittarius, the deep philosophical wisdom seeker, rules the liver, hips, thighs, pelvis, and femur. This pose strengthens the legs, thighs, hips, knees, and ankles.

◇◇◇◇◇◇◇◇◇◇◇◇◇◇◇◇◇◇◇◇◇◇◇◇◇◇◇◇◇◇◇◇◇◇◇

TRIANGLE POSE

» Stand straight. Separate your feet comfortably wide apart (about 3½ to 4 feet).

» Turn your right foot out 90 degrees and left foot in 15 degrees.

» Now align your right heel with the center of the arch of your left foot.

» Ensure that your feet are pressing the ground and the weight of your body is equally balanced on both feet.

» Inhale deeply and as you exhale, bend your body to the right, downward from the hips, keeping your waist straight, raising your left hand to come up in the air while lowering your right hand toward the floor. Keep both arms in a straight line.

» Rest your right hand on your shin, ankle, or the floor outside your right foot, whatever is possible without hyper-extending your waist. Stretch your left arm toward the ceiling, in line with the tops of your shoulders. Keep your head in a neutral position or turn it to the left, eyes gazing softly at the left palm.

» Ascertain that your body is bent sideways and not backward or forward. Your pelvis and chest are wide open.

» Stretch to your maximum and be steady. Keep taking in long, deep breaths. With each exhalation, relax the body more. Just be with your body and your breath.

» As you inhale, come back up to a sitting position, bring your arms down to your sides, and straighten your feet.

» Repeat the same on the other side.

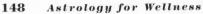

capricorn

Capricorn rules the bones, joints, knees, and teeth. Capricorns are determined and appreciate structure. This pose tones and roots the mind into the earth.

◇◇◇◇◇◇◇◇◇◇◇◇◇◇◇◇◇◇◇◇◇◇◇◇◇◇◇◇◇◇◇◇◇◇

MOUNTAIN POSE

» Stand straight with your feet together.

» Tighten your quadriceps muscles and lengthen your spine.

» Press your shoulders down, lengthen your neck, and rest your arms at your side, or bring them to the center of your chest.

» Feel a strong line of energy from your feet to the crown of your head, stretching your head toward the sky.

» Stay in the pose for a minute.

◇◇◇◇◇◇◇◇◇◇◇◇◇◇◇◇◇◇◇◇◇◇◇◇◇◇◇◇◇◇◇◇◇◇

aquarius

Aquarius rules the circulatory system, ankles, Achilles heels, calves, shins. Aquarians are the nonconformist, out-of-the-box thinkers with a humanitarian drive. This pose is excellent for improving blood circulation to the ankles and calves. Aquarians can be prone to cramps in the legs region.

◇◇◇◇◇◇◇◇◇◇◇◇◇◇◇◇◇◇◇◇◇◇◇◇◇

DOWNWARD FACING DOG

» Place your knees and hands on the floor, with your knees below your hips and your wrists in front of your shoulders.

» Your fingers should be spread wide with your middle finger pointing forward.

» Push your knees gently away from the floor, straightening your legs.

» Your knees should not be locked. With your sit bones lifted to the sky, try to move your heels down to touch the floor.

» Draw your shoulder blades down your back as your head rests between your arms.

» Stay in the pose for a minute.

◇◇◇◇◇◇◇◇◇◇◇◇◇◇◇◇◇◇◇◇◇◇◇◇◇

pisces

Pisces rules the feet and lymphatic system. They need a gentle type of yoga as they are sensitive souls—soft and caring personalities that can be prone to melancholy or escapism. This is a restorative pose that promotes relaxation, tranquility, insight, interconnectedness, and healthy emotional release.

◇◇◇◇◇◇◇◇◇◇◇◇◇◇◇◇◇◇◇◇◇◇◇◇◇◇◇◇◇◇◇◇◇◇◇

CHILD'S POSE

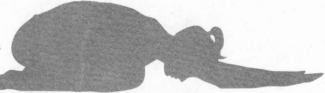

» Sit on your heels. Keeping your hips on your heels, bend forward and lower your forehead to the floor.

» Keep your arms alongside your body with hands on the floor, palms facing up. (If this is not comfortable, you can place one fist on top of the other and rest your forehead on them).

» Gently press your chest on your thighs.

» Hold.

» Slowly raise your abdomen, uncurling your spine vertebra by vertebra and come up to sit on your heels.

◇◇◇◇◇◇◇◇◇◇◇◇◇◇◇◇◇◇◇◇◇◇◇◇◇◇◇◇◇◇◇◇◇◇◇

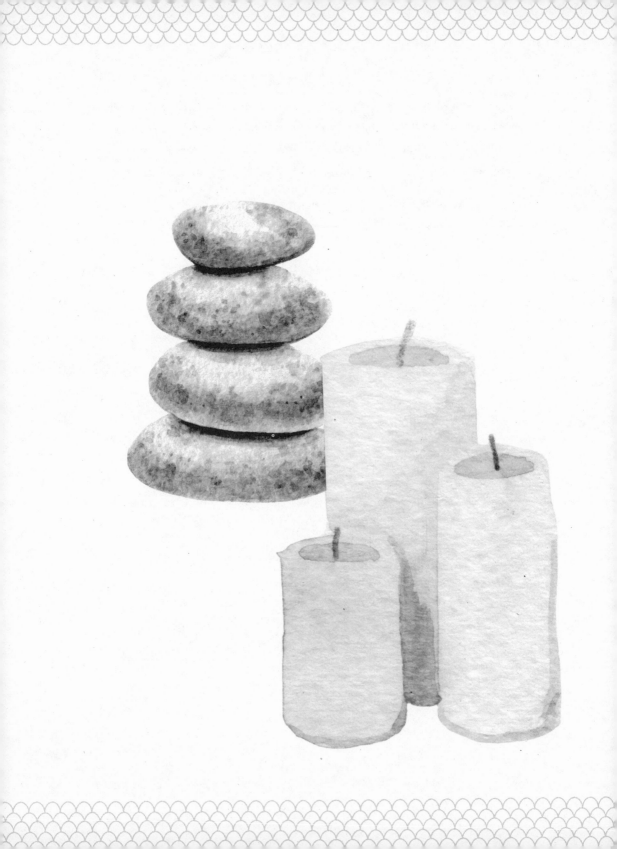

11

Mindful Meditations

FOR

Each Sign

We have designed these mindful meditations to guide you in dealing with the challenges of your Sun Sign. By sitting still, calming our breath, and watching our thoughts, we soon see the clarity of our real nature emerge. It shines through the haze of distraction and illuminates deeper levels of meaning and revelations, which can make us truly content. This is mindful meditation.

When most people think of meditation they imagine someone sitting cross-legged and chanting "Om" as a long, drawn out sound. This is the meditation we recommend for those born during the sign of Pisces. The goal of this kind of traditional meditation is to not allow the rational mind—with its insatiable desire to separate, name, count, and manipulate—to prevent us from directly experiencing our being.

Stilling the mind, diffusing our consciousness so we can experience universal mind, and focusing our awareness on the truth of our being require discipline and effort. Both traditional and our mindful meditations, also known as "waking meditations," challenge us to see through illusions and attachments and view them as different ways of looking at the same unifying truth.

For each meditation, sit comfortably in a place where you will not be disturbed and take a few deep and luxurious breaths before you begin to read and work with the mindfulness exercise for your Sun Sign. You might want to record yourself reading it aloud and play this back to yourself when doing an exercise requiring visualization.

We recommend that you explore the eleven other exercises for the other zodiac signs when you have mastered your own. As you do this, you are beginning to stretch your belief system. But the beliefs and habits you have created in the past have, symbolically, lives of their own, and like you, they want to continue to live. They are not just going to lie down and die. We cannot stress too many times how important it is to build mindfulness practices into daily routine, just as it is necessary to do physical exercise daily to the best of your ability to stay fit or get in better shape.

The only way to overcome really deep-seated beliefs about yourself and your world is through daily, patient practice. Otherwise, the rigidity that can sometimes plague even the most dedicated practitioner can not only limit growth but actually make people around you almost long for the return of your old ways. Mindfulness exercises can help you to become more aware of your thoughts and not allow them to just ramble on and on, meandering from one idle worry to the next.

aries:
FEAR MEDITATION

If you want to be free of irrational fears and phobias then you might want to take a few minutes each day to act "as if" you already are. You must tell yourself that you are cool, calm, and collected even if you know you are going to be in a situation that scares you, like a test, job interview, public speaking, or interacting with unpleasant people. Do not waste your time worrying that you might fail or that people will think you are foolish. Instead, take the time to do this exercise with the certain knowledge that it can help you.

Do some slow, deep breathing to relax yourself. Visualize yourself in the situation that you fear, but see yourself calm and successfully able to do what you know you can and want to do. See yourself happy to accomplish your goal. Tell yourself "I've gotten where I am because I am strong and can overcome anything I need to overcome. I have done this before. I don't have to be afraid. I am enjoying this."

When you have reprogrammed this way, you will be free of anxiety in the real situation because you have reinforced the experience as a positive one. Your unconscious mind does not know the difference between events actually experienced in normal waking consciousness and those experienced as strongly felt images, especially those experienced while you are in an alpha state.

As real as you can see it is as real as it can be. The more you see yourself as the strong person you are and build up your self-esteem, the better you will be able to face what life brings to you. You deserve happiness. By acting "as if," you are telling the very cells of your body that you already are.

taurus:

MANIFESTATION MEDITATION

Do some deep breathing to relax. In your mind's eye, picture stepping into an open car at the beginning of a tunnel. The walls of the tunnel may be natural rock, brick, tile, or any other surface you prefer. When you sit down in the car it begins to move through the tunnel at a comfortable speed. In the distance there is a light at the end of the tunnel, and as you move toward it you notice a sign above your head on the tunnel wall with the number twenty-two written on it. As you continue, always breathing slowly and deeply, you pass signs with the numbers twenty-one, twenty, nineteen, eighteen, seventeen, sixteen, fifteen, fourteen, thirteen, twelve, eleven, ten, nine, eight, seven, six, five, four, three, two, one.

You have reached the light at the end of the tunnel. You are now in a place where you and your unconscious mind will communicate. To do this, see yourself somewhere in a place where you can feel absolutely safe and at peace. This is the place you've always dreamed of being in. Or maybe it is a place that you actually visited once and had such a wonderful time that you have always wanted to go back again.

You decide where you are and what your special place of power is going to look like. You are there now. What do you see? Observe what comes into your mind without judgment. There is no right or wrong in your special place.

You may see yourself as if you were in a movie filmed in your special place of power or you may feel yourself in the scene so vividly that you can see and even smell your surroundings as if you were there—because (to your unconscious mind) you are there.

And now, as you see yourself vividly in your place of power, see and feel that you are happy, healthy, and more relaxed than you have ever felt before. See yourself doing what you've been longing to do. You may see yourself doing the job that you most want to be doing and being paid well for your work. You may see yourself with your ideal partner, someone who is treating you the way you want to be treated. Or you may see yourself looking the way you want to look and weighing the amount you want to weigh.

Let yourself feel really good about what you are seeing and feeling in your place of power. Let your unconscious mind know that this is the way you really want things to be. Make a friend of your unconscious mind and talk to it as a friend. Realize that it lives to help you get your life into the condition that you feel best about. Tell it how you want it to be as you show it the images that are real for you now in your special place of power. Linger there awhile, luxuriating in these pleasant sensations. Your unconscious mind now knows that this is what you want to experience and will now begin reprogramming itself to help you to bring these pleasant experiences into your daily life.

When you want to, leave your place of power by getting back into the car that brought you. But know that you can come back anytime you want to. Feel the car reenter the tunnel you came in from. Notice the numbers on the signs on the roof of the tunnel: one, two, three, four, five, six, seven, eight, nine, ten, eleven, twelve, thirteen, fourteen, fifteen, sixteen, seventeen, eighteen, nineteen, twenty, twenty-one, twenty-two. You're back. Slowly, open your eyes. You should feel relaxed and refreshed.

Notice how you felt about seeing yourself doing what you really want to be doing. Did you feel you deserved to get your wish? Did you believe that it was even possible? Gently remind yourself now and again, especially when you are in your place of power, that it is possible for you to get your wish and that you do deserve it. Being resistant to change is a natural part of the changing process and does not make you unworthy of getting your heart's desire. Although you may not yet be experiencing your life exactly the way you want it to be you must remember that you are worthy of having things the way you want them right now, just the way you are.

gemini:

WRITING MEDITATION

Writing not only connects the brain to the body in a deliberate and concentrated way but also making this "blueprint" of your life is a creative act, and creativity is another way to practice using your power over yourself and your life. If you can make your list and not have to worry about anyone finding it, be thankful and write that down as one of the items in your plus column.

Using a separate notebook, divide a piece of paper 8½ x 11 or larger, down the middle. On one side make a list of all the good things about your life. Head this column as *My Good Fortune*. It is important that you list a few of these things first. Come on, there must be some good things to be thankful for. I sometimes think that one of the reasons we all have problems is so other people can be thankful that their problems aren't as bad as ours. I certainly have a lot of trouble feeling sorry for myself when I remember the many people who are less fortunate than I am. Now, do you remember some good things to be thankful for?

Next, make a list of the things you want to change in your life. Head this column as *Things that I Will Change*. I hope you have enough paper, because in both your *Good Fortune* and *Change*, columns you should list everything you can think of. Take your time.

Beneath these two columns make a heading titled, *How I Want Things to Be*, and also divide that list into two columns. Label one column *Short-Term Goals* and the other column *Long-Term Goals*.

Short-term goals are things like "I will practice one of the exercises"; "I will love and forgive both myself and others before I go to sleep tonight"; "I will tell those I love how much I care about them today"; "I will organize my workspace"; "I will be aware of how my actions affect others";

"I will be aware of ___ , a habit whose origin I will soon understand"; "I will stop smoking/drinking/overeating for today and take it one day at a time"; and as many other ideas that you can think of that are goals to be remembered and attained every day.

Long-term goals are things like "I will stop smoking/drinking/overeating"; "I will look and feel great and weigh ___ pounds"; "I will earn my living by doing ___"; "I will meet and marry the partner of my dreams"; "I will attain financial security"; and as many other ideas as you can think of that are goals that you will reach by both the daily attainment of your short-term goals and the other changes that will result from your daily practice of the different metaphysical fitness exercises.

Always write, "I will," never "I'll" or "I will try"—you will accomplish your goals, both long- and short-term, because your will power will be getting stronger from being used day by day. Writing "I will" is a subtle yet powerful reminder to us that it is because of our will that our life is going to change.

Leave some space for things you think of later and then beneath that write down a list of *What I've Allowed to Stop Me*—all the things you think have prevented you from having things the way you want them. This part of the list is very important.

When you list your obstacles it will become apparent, sooner or later, that you can devise methods for dealing with them. No matter how out of your control these obstacles appear to be, you are always in control of your end of the equation and you can figure out how to change and adapt to reach the goals you have set for yourself.

What you have to do is explore every possibility you can think of. You must also use every means, both physical and metaphysical, at your disposal, along with the precious and hard-won knowledge we all gain from the mistakes we make along the way. Perseverance and concentration seem to be the only thing in common between every successful person I have ever met or read about.

Update this list every week or so. You will be surprised at how some of your short-term goals become incorporated into your life as new habits that will replace the ones you wanted to change. When you attain any of your long-term goals, I suggest that you reward yourself in some way and make a little ceremony out of crossing it off of your list.

cancer:
INSECURITY MEDITATION

The next time you feel insecure or doubt your ability to handle stress of any kind, imagine yourself as a five-year-old child and talk to yourself that way—the way you would comfort a frightened child—either in your head or out loud (if you are alone). If it helps, you may want to carry a picture of yourself as a child and talk to it. Tell this inner child that you love it and that everything is going to be all right.

Think about how you, as the loving parent, would nurture yourself as this scared, sensitive, and insecure child. You might say, "I know you are scared. Everyone gets scared sometimes. But it's okay. I'm here. I love you so very much. I'll protect you. Don't worry."

Don't just say it, feel it! Give your inner child the kind of unconditional love that a parent is supposed to give a child. Some people reserve this kind of love for their pets. Give your inner child the kind of love that accepts it just the way it is. Tell it that no matter what happens you will always love it.

If you have been angry with yourself, apologize to your inner child for scaring it and explain that you just lost your temper and now you feel much better. If you ever thought you were fat, ugly, or unattractive in any way, apologize and tell this child that it is pretty, handsome, and cute and that you love it. You can never tell your inner child too many times that you love it; that everything is going to be all right; and that it is a very good child. Children thrive on reassurance, and children of dysfunctional families—and that is unfortunately most of us—need as much reassurance and love as they can get.

It is unreasonable to expect our family and friends and the outside world to give us this kind of constant encouragement but we can and must supply it to ourselves. Little by little, you will develop more self-confidence with these self-nurturing techniques.

leo:
CREATIVITY MEDITATION

Having the intention to grow like a seed is at the heart of creativity.

The challenge to live life creatively is the challenge to recapture the sense of adventure, wonder, and playfulness that children—those seeds of infinite human possibility—naturally possess. Children see a situation and ask questions and make statements that can enable even adults who thought they knew everything about the situation to learn something completely new about it. At the heart of our book is the following warm-up exercise.

Although this exercise seems simple at first reading, if you actually try it, you will find it is incredibly powerful. Remember, to really and truly change your life, you must start from where you are, examine your situation, and take a chance on yourself by making all changes that suggest themselves. Play this little game and your reward will be a creative approach to life. Have a pad and a pen to journal your insights:

Look at your situation as if you were seeing it for the first time.

Do not assume you know it all, but question everything with the bravery of a child; without fearing that you will bring up answers you may not like.

Ask yourself, what is really going on?

How is it affecting you and the situation you want to change creatively?

If you could wave a magic wand and make anything happen, how would you want things to be?

What is preventing things from being that way, the way you'd like them to be?

What, if anything, can be done to effect the changes necessary to eliminate whatever is standing in your way?

See yourself doing what has to be done. Take note of what you see in your mind's eye and write it down.

If nothing can be done, why is that?

Isn't there some other way of doing it?

Is your desire to change really in your best interest?

If it is, and you are ready to do what is necessary, then do what pioneering imagery expert Gerald Epstein, MD, so creatively advises us to do: You must separate your intention from your attention. In other words, do not dwell on how you are going to surmount the obstacles presently in your way. Let your subconscious mind do its job without interference. You will be surprised when a creative flash of inspiration comes to you and gives you the solution about how to proceed.

virgo:
PERFECTIONIST MEDITATION

Have you ever been sure that you couldn't do something? Were you being too critical or perfectionistic, which caused you to procrastinate? I'll bet that, whatever it was, it didn't get done, at least not by you, until either you or somebody else convinced you that maybe you could do it after all. And then you did it!

Virgos can often be so focused on the minutia of a situation that they forget to examine the big picture. They can even forget that in the past they have overcome their perfectionism and done many things that they thought they could not do.

Let's hold the memory of this type of event for a moment. Remember a time when you believed you could not do something but you went ahead and tried anyway and did it! Remembering times like this can give us a boost of strength anytime and anywhere we need one. It sounds simple but it works.

What changed? The task to be done was the same. You were the same person—or were you? You changed what you believed you could do and so you were then able to do it. You changed your experience of your life! If you don't think that was a powerful thing you did, remember the many documented cases of people lifting incredibly heavy weights to rescue people trapped beneath them.

In the grip of powerful emotions, these "miraculous" heroines and heroes forgot they believed that they couldn't lift cars and collapsed walls and so they were able to lift them. When you lifted the "weight" of your restrictive belief in the "fact" that you couldn't do the task and did it, you rescued your true self from being crushed by your self-doubt and joined the ranks of the real super-people. As it is written in the Book of Tao, a beautifully simple ancient Chinese book of philosophy, " He who conquers others is strong. He who conquers himself is mighty."

libra:

BALANCING MEDITATION

The balancing meditation for Libras is designed to connect you to and balance your *chakras*, a word meaning "wheels," the seven energy centers distributed from the base of your spine to the crown of your head that are often seen as spinning colored energy vortexes by experienced meditators in their deepest sessions. The ups and downs of daily life can throw them off their natural course and leave you feeling disharmonious. Our meditation is designed to re-establish harmony.

Take a few deep breaths and get comfortable. Then close your eyes and visualize in your mind's eye the number one. Picture it a brilliant shade of red. Slowly breathe in that fiery red color for a count of six, hold it for a count of three, and then slowly breathe it out for a count of six.

As you pause in between breaths for a count of three, see the number two colored like an orange. Now breathe the orange color in for a count of six, hold it for a count of three, and breathe it out for a count of six.

As you pause between breaths see the number three as the color yellow. Breathe it in for a count of six, hold it in for a count of three, and breathe it out for a count of six.

As you pause between breaths see the number four as green, the color of healing. Slowly breathe it in, hold it, and breathe it out.

As you pause between breaths see the number five as a beautiful sky blue. Slowly breathe it in, hold it, and breathe it out.

As you pause between breaths see the number six as a deep indigo. Slowly breathe it in, hold it, and breathe it out.

As you pause between breaths see the number seven as a rich purple. Slowly breathe it in, hold it, and breathe it out.

You have now balanced your energy centers to feel relaxed and rejuvenated.

scorpio:

RELEASE MEDITATION

By feeling our power to control ourselves in the present moment we can extend that power to affect all areas of our experience.

If your present moment is a time of trauma or crisis, then where do you start? Right from where you are. Paramahansa Yogananda, author of the classic *Autobiography of a Yogi* and the first Indian master to bring the wisdom of Indian philosophy to the United States and Europe, wrote, "The time of failure is the best time to sow the seeds of success." By extension, the time of crisis is the best time to sow the seeds of better times to come.

You don't have to constantly mull over all of the problems you want to solve. Problems have a way of being there and ready to be dealt with when we are better prepared to deal with them, so let your problems get along without you for a little while.

Now the next thing you have to do is realize that it took a while for things to become the way they are and it's going to take a while for things to improve. But they will improve, you can bet on it! I can't stress enough how important it is for you to just believe that it is possible for you to change your experience of your life. You've got to be willing to admit into your belief system—what you believe to be true—that you can change your life. You can, period. It's not easy but it can be done. In fact, I'll bet you've already done it at some point in your life.

If you do the following invocation with a strong conviction, you should immediately feel the loving attention and support of the Great Spirit or whatever you choose to call the force that animates all life:

Close your eyes and breathe deeply. Feel your body relax. Breathe in through your nose while expanding your tummy, then blowing out slowly through your mouth. Do this six times. Visualize that you are a bird in an enclosed birdcage. You notice that the door is ajar. You can leave the cage of your own free will. Are you afraid to fly out, to be free, or is it more comfortable to stay inside?

Say these words, either out loud (if you are alone) or to yourself:

"Great Spirit, please help me. My anxieties crowd around me, seeking to trap me. My pain has a hold on me. Release me and grant me the freedom to fly and let go of all traps enclosing me."

Keep breathing deeply as you feel your spirit fly free into the light of Expansion and Liberation. Open your eyes and grant yourself a vacation from your pain.

sagittarius:
A MEAL MEDITATION

Nurturing, soothing, and stabilizing yourself and others is important in times of chaos and uncertainty. Being creative gives your mind a rest from stress and makes space for nourishing your soul and communion with spirit. True meditation allows you "to be" present, and being present while you're cooking and eating is a very fulfilling practice that will make you and others happy.

The Meal Meditation is about connecting to your inner self, acknowledging how beautiful, precious, and sacred life is. It is about your deep connection to the natural world that supports and sustains life. And it is about the need to stop, recalibrate, and focus attention on the many forms of nourishment, joy, and light that cooking and eating provide.

Here are eight tips to meditate on while you eat, cook, and entertain:

1. Use recipes that work for the season, your personality, and the appetites of your guests.

2. Make sure you have everything you need to prepare the meal: ingredients, equipment, utensils.

3. Take a few deep breaths and begin. Treat cooking as your sole focus while you are doing it.

4. Do one step and one task at a time before moving to the next one.

5. Incorporate prep work, cleanup, and even chanting into your cooking meditation practice.

6. Focus on the task at hand. Measure and marinate. Stir and add spice. Smell the aromas. Try to do this while not focusing on problems in the outside world or worries in your mind.

7. Make the table settings as special as the meal. Let your intuition and imagination guide you to color and arrangements. Flowers can lift your spirit.

8. Wash your hands. Light a candle that is in a safe and fireproof candleholder. Say a blessing. Sit down and enjoy your food, the textures and tastes, each bite, and your company. Inhale. Exhale. Let yourself be nourished and grateful.

Please note: Never leave a candle burning unattended.

capricorn:

RESPONSIBILITY MEDITATION

You can usually spot areas of your life that need changing because they are sources of pain, suffering, and sometimes, a good deal of boredom for you or for those who are close to you and who care about you. Things related to these areas don't seem to work well for you, no matter how hard you try. You may even be literally "sick and tired" from "beating your head against the wall."

But our pain is also a spotlight shining on the areas of our life where work is needed. And just like that spotlight, we are going to concentrate our light—the light of our awareness—on those painful areas because that is the kind of light that can heal them.

As you honestly confront those areas of your life that need work, it is very important that you take some of the responsibility for what has happened to you in the past. Taking responsibility for your life is an admission that you have power over what happens to you.

And so you must sit up and take notice of your situation. Where are you? What is the problem? What must be done to correct it? You must focus on the present moment because the present is the only place where your power is concentrated. The past is beyond your control and the future is . . . well, in the future. But you can affect the future by living and acting in the present moment. By feeling your power to control yourself in the present moment you can extend that power to affect all areas of your experience.

aquarius:

FREEDOM MEDITATION

When we get stressed out, maxed out, and overwhelmed, we move into lower function—anger, aggravation, fear, and low self-esteem. If we consciously turn within and calm ourselves with positive affirmations, meditations, and visualizations, we can move our assimilating abilities "up" so we can better cope and tap into a healthy clear flow of energy that frees our circuits from being clogged. This process helps us feel in control of our destiny.

Mindfulness is the main idea of meditation—to be aware of our thoughts and state of mind. That is the only way we can really rid ourselves of things that become negative patterns that fester and hurt us and hurt our psyches.

Worry happens when analysis ceases to be scientific and we become attached mentally and emotionally to knowing that there will or will not be a particular outcome. We become impatient and irrational because only experience over time will reveal whether what we believe will happen will, indeed, happen.

When you are aware of being in tune with the universe, you know then that everything has its own seasons, rhythms, and cycles. However, in our dimensional world these things not only come around in full circle but are part of a spiral carrying us ever onward and upward in our evolution and growth.

Here's an idea: Why not, if only for a day, avoid worrying about what you think is wrong or is going to go wrong? Even if you are in dire straits, and I've been there, worrying will not help you now. Concentrate on staying positive and grateful and being open to new possibilities and opportunities. If you worry, you will not see as clearly your path to obtaining a reasonable amount of what you to consider success.

Rough times are times when little things can be very important. Subtle hints of how to behave and where to go are easily overwhelmed by worrying about impending problems that may or may not actually come into being.

We each bring experiences into our life to teach us the lessons we would like to learn. It is up to you to decide what you can learn from your present experience. If you spend your precious time thinking about what you are upset about, you are wasting time that could otherwise be spent helping you move into a better probable future.

Worry is based on our attachment to wanting to know how things will turn out. The way to balance worry is first to acknowledge that it is based on our natural desire to avoid pain. Worry is like a well-meaning friend who keeps picking everything apart to try to make it better, yet if that friend is allowed to go on and on, what he or she ends up with is a pile of picked-apart pieces of a whole that does not work anymore.

If you can't take even a one-day vacation from worry, then sit comfortably and simply keep repeating the words "no worries" until you start to allow yourself to have no worries for a few minutes. After you do that, you can again let worry have its say and thank it for its trouble. In this way, worries are allowed to serve their legitimate purpose and you will not feel bad every time you notice you are worrying. Try to be in the moment by practicing meditation, breathing, and mindfulness.

pisces:
SENSITIVITY MEDITATION

One of the reasons many people seem to be becoming insensitive to human suffering is because of the large amounts of it, both real and theatrical, that can be seen every minute of every day in living color right in our living rooms. After long exposure, our unconscious mind numbs us to the natural feelings evoked by watching others in pain.

Remember that your unconscious mind responds to strongly felt images and feelings caused by your experiences and your beliefs about your experiences. Your unconscious mind is also the source of your instinctual responses.

Something very important to remember is that your unconscious mind responds to the movie and to scenes you watch in exactly the same way as it responds to the situations you actually see in real life. It takes your reactions seriously and programs itself to accomplish your desires of either repeating a strongly felt pleasurable experience or protecting you from any unpleasant experiences.

For this reason you should try to be aware of the images you are sending to your unconscious mind by the television shows and movies that you watch. At the very least, these images can cause quite a bit of confusion unless you are aware of what you are doing and communicate it to your unconscious mind through the following meditation, a practice that has stood the test of thousands of years and countless practitioners in its ability to counteract the effects of daily life on our sensitive natures.

Sit comfortably in a place where you will not be disturbed for at least five minutes. Take three deep breaths in and then out. When you release the third breath, use it to say the sound *Om* so that you use the entire breath you are releasing to do so. *Om* is an ancient and sacred sound in Hinduism, Buddhism, and Jainism. Its use in our meditation is designed to take us beyond words, beyond form, and beyond the reach of anything and everything that distracts us from remembering the scientifically proven fact that we are all one. Einstein's theory of $E=mc^2$ proved that all matter is energy. Chanting *Om* while breathing in and out and focusing on nothing else but the sound can help us cleanse our sensitive nature.

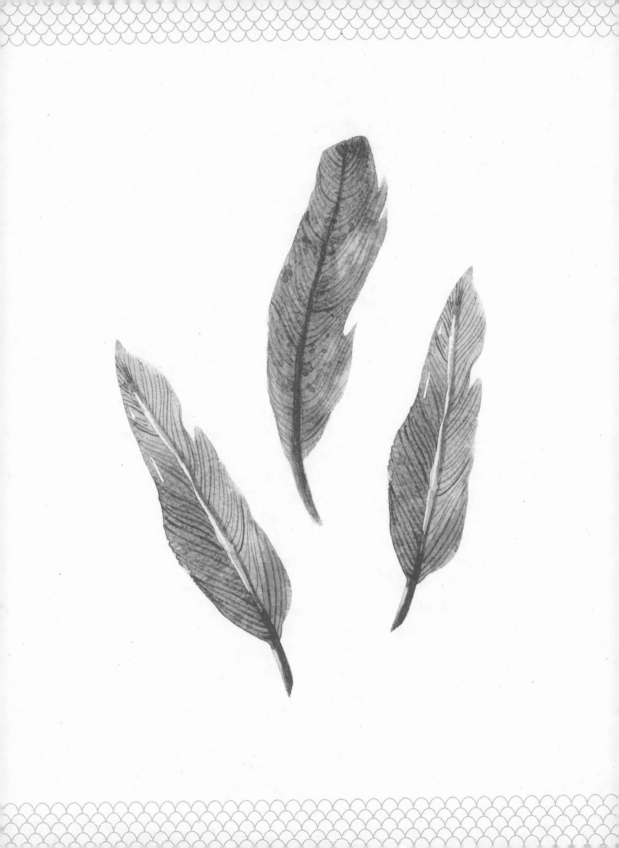

12

Breathing Affirmations

FOR

Each Sign

We are going to learn how to use our breathing combined with affirmations to attain the very important goal of relaxation. It is well known that the best way to learn anything is to be in a state of relaxed attention while learning. Otherwise, tension and anxiety can prevent even the most dedicated students from absorbing and retaining anywhere near the knowledge they could if they were relaxed.

Our breathing, just like the way we live our life, can be done in either an unconscious fashion that will just keep us alive or in a conscious fashion that will actually enable us to control our mind and body, bringing them into natural harmony with our spirit.

Our breathing is the most obvious example of how our mind can influence our body. Our every mood is unintentionally reflected in our manner of breathing. If we are anxious or agitated, we tend to breathe in a shallow but rapid manner, physically mirroring our restricted or agitated state. Our breathing is calm when we are calm and it is the deepest and the slowest when we are the most relaxed as when we are sleeping.

It has been proven that if you force your facial muscles to make yourself smile, even when you are sad, you will start to feel happier. Your body will also start showing the many beneficial results that would normally occur if your smile had been caused by a pleasurable thought or experience. In a similar manner, since our breathing is the only one of our internal processes that we can easily exert direct conscious control over, we can put ourselves into a relaxed state by breathing the way we do when we are most relaxed, i.e., slowly and deeply.

When you do your breathing exercises on a regular, daily basis, they can have many life-changing effects. All they require is a little concentration. Many times we forget to listen to the inner voice that connects us to the divine. When we breathe consciously, with love and trust, we regain our connection to that divine spark of knowing and being.

Imagination gives us the ability to create a better body and a better world for that body to exist in. Visualization is seeing a picture of what you are trying to achieve in your mind to help you create it in reality. Imagining or remembering a frightening event can tense you. Imagining a beautiful scenario with all of your five senses can counter the negative effects of stress by putting you in the state of relaxed concentration. This is "the zone" in which optimum learning, analysis, and planning can take place.

BASIC BREATHING EXERCISE:

Sit comfortably in a place where you know you won't be disturbed. If you are wearing tight or restrictive clothes, loosen them.

Breathe in slowly through your nose and picture in your mind's eye your diaphragm curving downward as your lower lungs fill with life-giving air and your stomach pushes out slightly like an expanding balloon. Continue to breathe in and let the air fill the middle of your lungs as you expand your rib cage. Complete your inhalation by lifting your chest (not your shoulders) as you fill the top of your lungs. While you are inhaling you should be counting from one to six.

If you are comfortable doing this, hold your breath for a count of three—half as long as it took you to inhale. When you first start doing this exercise you may not feel comfortable holding your breath at all. At first try holding your breath for one second before exhaling. Do it this way until you are comfortable and feel that you can try holding your breath for two seconds before exhaling. Only do what you feel comfortable doing. You can gradually increase the time, always making sure that you are not straining yourself or hyperventilating. Under no circumstances should you hold your breath in between inhaling and exhaling for longer than three seconds for the first few months of doing this exercise.

Now exhale through your mouth for a count of as long as it took you to inhale. Start your exhalation by slowly pulling in your stomach as you picture your diaphragm curving up, pushing the air up and out of your lungs. Continue to exhale as you contract your rib cage and lower your chest.

Wait as long as you are comfortable before starting your next breath. At first you may not be able to wait at all and that is perfectly fine. As you get used to this exercise you may be able to gradually increase the time you can comfortably wait between breaths to a count of six—as long as the time it takes to inhale and exhale. You will then be able to reach an even deeper level of relaxation.

Continue to breathe this way for a few minutes. At first you will be a bit self-conscious as you try to get the breathing right but that feeling will pass. When you are comfortable with this exercise and no longer have to concentrate so single-mindedly on the mechanics of it you might find that your mind will start to occupy itself with its usual stream of consciousness. When you catch yourself doing that, just notice each thought in a detached manner, let it go without exploring it any further, and go back to focusing on your breathing.

After you have relaxed and done the breathing exercise for your Sun Sign, you will be better prepared to deal with any or all distracting matters.

These twelve astro-specific breathing affirmation rituals can be done when you are anxious, tense, or angry or experiencing great stress or before you are going to have to pay close attention to some matter, either something you want to learn or must remember.

Just as we were able to change how we feel by taking control of our breath, our breathing rituals help prepare us to take control of our lives.

ARIES

The child you were still lives within you and needs to play and feel secure. "I breathe in the innocence of a child's mind that sees all things as if for the first time. I am filled with childlike joy and zest for life. I breathe out the illusion of age."

TAURUS

Focus and clarity comes from the practice of being one-pointed in your attention.

"I breathe in the discipline to make strengthening my body, mind, and spirit an enjoyable daily ritual. I am filled with determination. I breathe out procrastination and distraction."

GEMINI

Much can be learned from everyone and everything, even the "nets" that try to snare us.

"I breathe in the wisdom that the flow of nature is offering me. I am filled with the desire to learn all I can about life and about my place in it. I breathe out ignorance."

CANCER

Make your home base secure and you will feel comfortable no matter where you go.

"I breathe in the feeling that I am safe and protected. I am filled with self-confidence enabling me to love and accept others even more. I breathe out insecurity."

LEO

Creativity enables us to artfully address life's challenges.

"I breathe in the energy to create and renew my body and soul. I am filled with the ability to learn useful disciplines that can help me heal my world. I breathe out my fear of being judged."

VIRGO

Everything in moderation, nothing in excess; this is the way to lead a life of quality and meaning.

"I breathe in the perfection of the earth, the water, and the sky. I am filled with nature's grand design. I breathe out my self-destructive tendencies."

LIBRA

Beauty is found in the exchange of love between all beings.

"I breathe in the beautiful colors, fragrances, and forms around me. I am filled with the beauty that is my birthright. I breathe out the critic's voice that says things are not perfect."

SCORPIO

Each time we change ourselves, the whole world is changed.

"I breathe in the ability to see what is working in my life and what needs to be changed. I am filled with the courage and excitement that change brings. I breathe out my fear of letting go."

SAGITTARIUS

Every step of life's journey is an important adventure.

"I breathe in the pleasure and increased awareness that accompanies my travels. I am filled with infinite energy that animates my life and everything around me. I breathe out fear of newness."

CAPRICORN

When life overwhelms us, it is time to get outside and touch the earth to ground ourselves, reestablishing our essential unity with nature.

"I breathe in the comfort of Mother Earth. I am filled with a connection to Earth's center. I breathe out anxiety."

AQUARIUS

A caring friend is worth more than any worldly possessions.

"I breathe in the loving friendship that makes life's struggles bearable. I am filled with love, light, and laughter to be shared with my friends. I breathe out all loneliness and distrust."

PISCES

When we awaken to our ability to create our own reality, all our dreams are possible.

"I breathe in the manifestation of my hopes and wishes. I am filled with the knowledge that my dreams can come true. I breathe out doubt and despair."

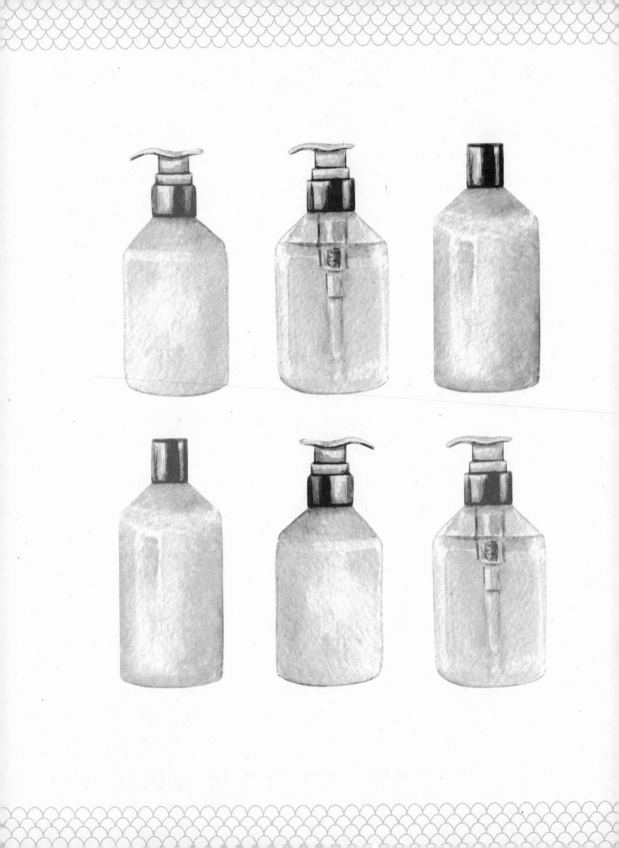

13

Beauty Tips

FOR

Each Sign

Beauty is often stated as being in the eye of the beholder. But there is also a connection between beauty and wellness. And a connection between one's mind and body is recognized as an important aspect of beauty and skin care. When we are anxious, unhappy, or tired, our skin loses its glow and energy. Our skin mirrors our life. Here we address some beauty tips through the lens of the zodiac.

ARIES

The speed of the beauty regime is important. You are too energetic to tie yourself down to one beauty product or one way of treating your skin. You like to try new things. You want variety—different nourishing facial masks are perfect for Aries as this sign rules the face and head, and they calm you down for a minute. It takes a fast-acting mask to keep up with your speed. You might prefer no parabens, gluten free, and fragrance free.

TAURUS

You like to stick to a system. You become rather fixed in your habits and you cannot tolerate deviation from your system: first cleanser, then toner, then serum, then moisturizer, then eye cream. Don't forget neck cream! You could benefit from changing up your routine a bit. You tend to accumulate skin, hair, makeup, and nail tools and buy a lot as you are in love with beauty.

GEMINI

Geminis are influenced by influencers. To you, beauty is a game. You long to capture the perfect prize that eludes your grasp: a product that has perfect dual functions and works for both day and night, cheeks and lips, two functions in one. Once you find something you love, you have a genius for sharing information. You would like airbrushed makeup or fun treatments that bubble or fizz.

CANCER

You tend to buy a product if it touches you emotionally. You form a gut response to the vibrations of color, and the colors and designs in beauty packaging stimulate you. Laborsaving devices, such as skin exfoliating gadgets, also have an appeal to you; and you fill your medicine cabinet with them—products with pearl or that work for nighttime appeal. Also, cruelty-free beauty products are important to you.

LEO

Drama is key. You love to be on parade and are always ready for "showtime." A date without low lights, glam makeup, and good music would be as inspiring as a salad without dressing. You go out of your way to discover the best high-end beauty products wherever and whenever they are to be found. You may be attracted to products that shimmer and glow and that make you feel like you "shine."

VIRGO

Discrimination is your greatest skill. You are a perfectionist, and because of this faculty for minute analysis, you are very picky with what you purchase or put on your face. You are interested in organic products with herbal elements. You are seldom fooled by miracle claims because your keen mental perception enables you to detect a lie. Handmade soaps and natural shampoos that don't contain chemical preservatives would suit.

LIBRA

You have an appreciation for all beautifying agents and items. Your appreciation of beauty makes you seek products that will always remain useable, beneficial, and attractive and that help you appear to be unmarred by wear and tear. Dependability is important to you. You are faithful to your beauty regime and loyal to your brands. They both must smooth and soothe! When shopping, you have an excellent sense of ethical and material values. The pH level of the skin refers to how acidic or alkaline it is. Try skin care systems that address and balance the pH of your skin.

SCORPIO

Scorpio is all about passion. You tend to be devoted to (and obsessed by!) one special chosen beauty product at a time. You can become a veritable tornado of beautification. Your intense observational nature causes you to exaggerate minor faults and flaws, and you are always searching for solutions. Let your heart rule when buying—you love the lavish and luxurious. You might like a jade roller—a traditional Chinese beauty product.

SAGITTARIUS

You plunge into beauty care with zeal. Your tastes are dictated by your fervor for nature or your devotion to the outdoors. You do not hesitate to change your mind when you find something more alluring. When shopping, at heart you are a hunter who enjoys the thrill of pursuit. A very versatile, ingenious product could keep you interested—something waterproof or mineral based, something that supports and restores your skin to its natural defenses.

CAPRICORN

Usefulness is important to a Capricorn. You consider self-care important, and are conscientious in your duties to your skin's health. Nevertheless, you are so economical that you will shop for the lesser-priced merchandise if you believe it will deliver the same results. Logic is an outstanding trait of your personality. So whether you're fighting wrinkles, zits, or sunspots, you look for efficiency in your beauty products.

AQUARIUS

Apply with skill. When others must struggle and study for years to attain beauty applications, techniques, and secrets, you acquire knowledge, information, and skills with seeming unconsciousness. You are ultramodern in your outlook and may be said to be ahead of the times so you are always

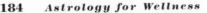

looking for cutting edge products: something breakthrough, microfine, or detoxifying. Since you cannot be restricted in any way, goals for your skin change and evolve, helping you to determine a treatment at any given moment. You tend to have an arsenal of approaches ready.

PISCES

Because you are a dreamer, sometimes you are impractically romantic when it comes to beauty. The fickle side of your nature might lead you into temptation, but the innate sense of the true, which you have, would not tolerate such indulgence for long. Be guided by your intuitional love for the finest and you won't be disappointed. Algae make a great natural moisturizer that improves skin's barrier function and helps it retain water. Also, you would love an eye palette with colors of the rainbow.

14

Healing Colors

FOR

Each Sign

Color is a powerful force, the visible manifestation of atomic vibration and energy absorption. Using color properly can improve your appearance, your home life, and your place of business. The right color promotes the vibrations that can enhance moods, set the tone for meetings of all kinds, and accent natural beauty in a number of magical ways. Without color, the world is a drab place, indeed. With it, all things are possible.

Color is vibration, the basic energy form underlying all of creation. Color is an essential ingredient in our daily environment. Not only does it communicate emotion and create a mood, but also it has the power to affect our energy levels. In this way, seeing a color and experiencing a color are virtually inseparable, because much of what is seen is also felt. People react to colors, because they evoke personal emotions and experiences.

What are your lucky astro colors? If you know, that's great! Make use of "our colors" in every possible way. When wearing fashions made of them, you will be more confident in yourself than when arrayed in something else. You will get more work done and it will be better work. Not only should you wear your astro colors, but it is a good idea to surround yourself with them. You intuitively select colors that will have a positive healing effect for you.

Meditate on a specific color in order to get a benefit from it. Clear your mind, take a few deep breaths, and stare at an object in the color you have chosen. Breathe in the color until you can feel it seep into your skin and deep inside you. Repeat this ritual whenever you feel as if you need a psychic "color infusion" in order to bring healing, happiness, prosperity, or any other good thing into your life.

ARIES: REDS (ALL SHADES)

Red signifies confidence and courage. It inspires boldness in thought and deed. A strong awareness of the physical body is indicated. There can sometimes be so much passion in its energy that when it is displayed it can be perceived as aggression. Red can be used to strengthen the body and to promote will power and courage. Wear red to stimulate vitality.

A simple spell for red: To inspire a sense of bravery, wear a red accessory. Even if the color is not immediately visible to anyone else (a piece of lingerie, a handkerchief, a piece of red construction paper folded in a purse

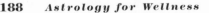

or wallet), you will know that you have this splash of red and will feel more courageous as a result.

TAURUS: SPRING GREEN, PINK

Pink is the color of personal happiness. This lively yet gentle shade reflects optimism, a youthful attitude, and the ability to take chances. It signifies romance. It has the ability to bring a fresh perspective to any endeavor. Pink can be used to promote self-esteem. Wear pink to welcome joy and beauty. Spring green says growth, balance, harmony.

A simple spell for pink: Everyone needs a little of this color in their life. Create a "pink corner" in your bedroom or bathroom. Do this by filling a shallow glass bowl with a variety of pink objects: stones, shells, even candy. Whenever you feel you need a fresh or more youthful perspective on matters, visit your pink corner and run your hands over the items. Your point of view will be refreshed and updated.

GEMINI: YELLOW, MULTICOLOR

The color yellow signifies cheerfulness, optimism, and bright ideas. It is a happy and energetic color that reflects mental acuity and communication. It is also a celebration of sunny days. Yellow energy is related to the ability to perceive and understand.

A simple spell for yellow: To create a feeling of confidence and happiness, wear yellow-gold jewelry to an event. If you are feeling worn-out or tired in the evening hours when the Sun has gone to sleep, sit under a lamp with your eyes closed. The warmth and light that permeate your closed lids will help you to concentrate on the power and promise of tomorrow's sunrise.

CANCER: SILVER, MAUVE, GRAY

Gray represents the middle ground, neither completely positive nor completely negative. Gray is used in color therapy to absorb unwanted energy from the body. Emotionally, it symbolizes a willingness to comply, to be purposefully isolated in order to find a quiet and balancing energy. Silver and mauve are Moon colors that help guide our intuition to make the best decisions.

A simple spell for gray: When meditating, picture your mind as a gray screen where messages will appear. Because gray has a restful and therapeutic affect, it will soothe your consciousness, making it easier for messages to come.

LEO: GOLD, ORANGE

Orange is a joyous color, representing vibrant energy and intellectual curiosity. It is the color of surprise and enthusiasm. It has a sense of humor; wearing a bit of orange can bring smiles and a sense of optimism, stimulate creativity and mental quickness and an ability to adjust to changes. Wearing orange during times of stress can help to balance your emotions.

A simple spell for orange: Keep a bowl of oranges on the table as a focal point in the morning. Their scent and bright color are exhilarating. Like the glass of orange juice it represents, it will start your day off right! To promote and facilitate learning a new subject, use an orange bookmark.

VIRGO: TAN, SAGE

Classic and understated, tan suggests the path of moderation, relaxation, undemanding energy, and neutrality. While it may be seen as representing a conservative attitude, its energy signifies dependability, caring, and common sense. Sage green is a color that communicates peace and growth and speaks of nature's wisdom.

A simple spell for tan: Take a cup of sand from your favorite beach and sift out the impurities. Then put the clean sand in a decorative bowl and keep it on your bedside table. Each night before going to sleep, cup a palmful of the sand, then open your fingers and let it drain back into the bowl as you say, "May my choices and opportunities be as numberless as these grains of sand." After a month, recycle the sand and replace it with a fresh supply.

LIBRA: LIGHT BLUE, ROYAL BLUE, WHITE

All shades of blue will help to make easier communications, whether they are with yourself or others. Blue symbolizes peace and emotional tranquility. It also inspires mental control, creativity, and clarity. Blue has a pacifying effect. It symbolizes the sky, the shielding dome above our heads and, therefore, represents boundless potential and opportunities. White is the emblem of innocence and purity and denotes spiritual authority.

A simple spell for blue: Whenever you are feeling stressed, put on a piece of blue clothing. Avoid dark or navy blue, because the lighter the shade of blue you choose, the more comforted and lighthearted you will feel. Meditating with a blue candle before bedtime promotes restful sleep.

SCORPIO: MAGENTA, MAROON

Magenta is the flag for innovative, strong-willed, imaginative, artistic, and creative individuals. It has the qualities of red, plus empathy; it is a mixture of passion and compassion. Magenta is ideal for rituals to secure ambitions and financial rewards. The maroon color is often used to aid confidence, courage, strength, warmth, and beauty.

A simple spell for magenta: To lift the vibe of your environment, put a sprig of the fuchsia plant into a bud vase. Keep it in the room where you spend a great deal of your time. An object of this color is favorable to use when attempting to make contact with the spirit world.

SAGITTARIUS: PURPLE (ALL SHADES)

Purple denotes power, authority, and psychic strength. In a metaphysical sense, purple energy connects us to our spiritual guidance, wisdom, and inner strength. Purple is a color of transformation, combating fear and resistance to change. Purple is used for meditation and to sharpen psychic awareness and connection with Higher Self and to increase imagination and inspiration.

A simple spell for purple: Tape a decorative purple embellishment to your mirror, or drape a purple shawl or throw over a chair. The presence of this vibrant color in your everyday life will remind you to live in the here and now, even while embracing spiritual truths.

CAPRICORN: BLACK, DARK BROWN, GREEN

Brown denotes practicality, simplicity, humility, and purposefulness. It is the ultimate earth tone, reflective of nature, as is green. Black is not actually a color but the absence of color. It can be off-putting because of its intensity, but it is actually comforting, protective, and mysterious. It is good for banishing negativity in oneself or fighting negativity from an outside source. On the practical level, black represents seriousness and commitment to an idea or principle—a total absorption with a cause.

A simple spell for black: Those drawn to black may be intractable and impervious to change. In order to combat this, perform the following ritual. On your altar or another safe area, place three candles—black, gray or silver, and white—side by side in fireproof candleholders. Each day light one of them, in order of their placement. By lighting the black candle only every third day, your subconscious mind will become subtly accustomed to change.

Please note: Never leave a candle burning unattended.

AQUARIUS: ELECTRIC BLUE, INDIGO, ULTRAVIOLET

Indigo is the color of spiritual awakening and awareness. It is an imaginative, intuitive, and mystical shade. It inspires sensitivity to beauty, harmony, and compassion for others as well as promoting lucid dreams and dream skills such as problem-solving. Ultraviolet energy strengthens intuition and connects us to a higher spiritual realm. Its subtle vibration can be useful in ESP such as telepathy, clairvoyance, and even astral projection.

A simple spell for indigo: If you have a special meditation area in your house or apartment, keep an indigo object ever present in this area. A scarf, a pillow, or a decorative object will call up indigo energy whenever you need to tap into its special power.

PISCES: LAVENDER, AQUA

Lavender is the color of spiritual healing, dispelling sadness, loneliness, and mental confusion. It is a good color for use on a ceremonial altar or in a room where meditation and rituals are practiced. Aqua is a serene yet uplifting color. Aqua promotes clear communication, honesty, openness, and the need to join together with others. It represents the ability to transform, just as water turns to ice and the cycle repeats.

A simple spell for lavender: If you are a seeker after truth and are traveling on a spiritual path, a sprig of lavender or some lavender-scented oil can be a reminder to stay centered and focused on your quest. Keeping track of your dreams in a lavender-colored notebook or diary is also a reminder of the importance of your spiritual search.

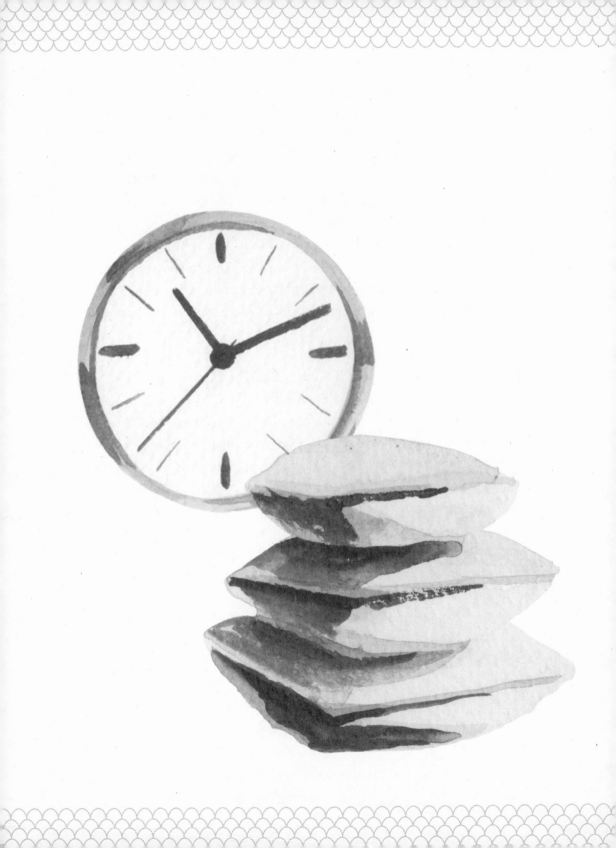

15

Sleep Advice

FOR

Each Sign

GO-TO-SLEEP EXERCISE:

Each night, before you go to sleep try to forgive those who have wronged you in your life. Start with yourself.

Forgive yourself for a mistake that you made that you would forgive in someone else if they had done the same thing. It is amazing how many of the things we think are so bad about ourselves are things we would not find so very terrible in those we like. We must like and love ourselves if we are to be able to feel and accept the love of others.

Many religious teachings whose goal it is to keep us from being overly proud and putting ourselves above their concept of God have gone overboard and instead taught children not to love, trust, and forgive themselves. This is a shame. We must now return to a more balanced view of ourselves that includes self-love, trust, and forgiveness. Perhaps it is our belief that we are all original sinners—imperfect and evil in the sight of God—that has allowed so many of us to do such horrible things to ourselves and each other. By forgiving ourselves we are taking the first step back to loving ourselves.

Continue to forgive yourself for all of the things that you have not been forgiving yourself for. Eventually you are going to come to something you have done that you cannot forgive yourself for. At that point don't push yourself but go on to forgive those who have wronged you. Start with your parents.

Picture your mother as a little girl about five or six years old. See her as a child not very different from your own inner child—scared, wanting love but unsure about how to get love in such a big and overwhelming world. Pick her up and comfort her. Wipe the tears from her eyes and tell her that you love her and that you will always be there when she needs you. That little girl needed love and forgiveness then just as she needs it now.

Realize that she was a younger person when she gave birth to you and that, though she wanted to do only the right things for you, she was suffering from the mistakes of her own life and of her own parents who were also only human beings. See her holding you after your birth and feel the love she had for you.

If she was not around after your birth or didn't treat you well, know that she wanted to be but fate had other plans for both of you. Now you are who you are, and if she had been around, you would not be who you are. Forgive your mother for all the human mistakes she made. Try to feel your forgiveness clean your heart and lungs of any grief they may have been holding. See your heart turn brightly golden and your lungs pink and healthy-looking, as the tarnish of unforgiveness is removed from them.

Now see your father as a little boy about five or six years old. See him as a child not very different from your own inner child, scared, wanting love but unsure about how to get love in such a big and overwhelming world. Pick him up and comfort him. Wipe the tears from his eyes and tell him that you love him and that you will always be there when he needs you. That little boy needed love and forgiveness then just as he needs it now.

Realize that he was a younger person when he fathered you and that, though he wanted to do only the right things for you, he was suffering from the mistakes of his own life and of his own parents who were also only human beings. See him holding you after your birth and feel the love he had for you.

If he was not around after your birth or didn't treat you well, know that he wanted to be but fate had other plans for both of you. Now you are who you are, and if he had been around or treated you differently, you would not be who you are. Forgive your father for all the human mistakes he made. Try to feel your forgiveness clean your heart and lungs of any grief they might have been holding. See your heart turn brightly golden and your lungs pink and healthy-looking, as the tarnish is removed from them.

Now forgive anyone who might have wronged you or anyone else you haven't forgiven in the past. You will occasionally think of someone who you can't bring yourself to forgive. You will be amazed at how often these people will be guilty of the very same thing that you cannot forgive yourself for. Try

forgiving both yourself and these other people for the things you have trouble forgiving. It is really true that as the Bible says, "Lest ye forgive, ye shall
not be forgiven." If you can forgive, you most assuredly will be forgiven. And
you will fall asleep when you want to.

comforters for each sign

ARIES

Aries is always on the go moving forward, and the only things that will help
Aries fall asleep are either total exhaustion or having the head, neck, and
face (gently) massaged. They don't like to wait, so they would want a comforter that warms them up fast, not necessarily an electric comforter but
something made out of a material like goose down that captures all their
body heat. It should also be thin enough as to be easy to move a limb or two
out of it because Aries hates to feel trapped. Another approach would be to
rest on a BioMat® or something similar, a pad that heats amethyst crystals
and black tourmaline and generates far-infrared light waves, heating you so
effectively from the inside out when you lie on it, you need little more than
a sheet as a cover. For sleeping, use a low-heat setting; the hotter settings are
great for shorter detox sessions.

TAURUS

What helps a Taurus fall asleep is to have a great meal followed by an
appreciation of the accomplishments of the day. Then to be in a beautifully
appointed room with a large, sumptuous bed to match, surrounded by some
of the wonderful pieces of their various collections and reminders of their
many triumphs over obstacles in their path. Their comforter would have to

be of the finest materials, as soft and luxurious as possible, and preferably thick and substantial. It could weigh more than any other sign would want a comforter to weigh.

GEMINI

A Gemini's mind is always acquiring and processing information, seeing two or more sides of a given situation. Their aversion to being bored can be an impediment to sleep because calming down to a resting state can seem similar to being bored. They need to blend calming down with surrender to the coming exciting experience of their dream world. Their comforter needs to be lightweight, even in cold weather. Actually, they would need to have two comforters so they could have enough choices as to how to regulate the temperature.

CANCER

Cancerians need to feel that the people they care about are safe and sound, and if this isn't true, falling asleep can be difficult. They need to visualize these people enveloped in their love and protection and that of whatever Higher Power they feel comfortable with. Of course, if small children are involved, no matter what sign you are, exhaustion will override whatever impediments there are to sleep. Cancerians need a comforter that makes them feel a connection to their past, perhaps a quilt that has been made by a relative and handed down or one that looks like it is from a time they feel connected to.

LEO

Leos sleep when Leos want to sleep, just like the lion that is the symbol of their zodiac sign. Going to sleep will be an event worthy of commentary, just like everything else they do, though they are not too fond of dreams because they cannot control them. It's waking up that is the issue for Leos; they have a tendency to want to stay in bed because that shows the world that no one tells them what to do. Obviously, this can be a problem for Leos who are salaried employees on a time clock. They need a comforter that makes a statement of grandeur in some way. It cannot be in muted colors or an understated pattern. Think "Napoleon's Comforter," and you'll be getting warm, or something resembling a stage set.

VIRGO

Virgos, like Geminis, have minds that are always going, but when Geminis are processing information, Virgos are worrying about the consequences of just about everything. To go to sleep they can benefit from my proven technique. Repeat slowly five times while breathing calmly and evenly and realizing the truth of the words, "I am not my name, I'm a spirit traveling onward." Then repeat slowly five times, "I am not what I do for a living, I'm a spirit traveling onward." They're usually asleep by the fourth time. Virgos need a comforter that has a pattern composed of small sections, the smaller the better. A crazy quilt would be good, though I think that would be better for a Cancer.

LIBRA

Libras seek harmony and if they don't get it, there are going to be consequences; so if the day was fraught with disharmony in any way they might have trouble falling asleep. They need to rise above any and all situations, as if they are an eagle soaring high over the world, and see that there is harmony even in the seeming disharmony of everyday life, and in the scheme of things, the problems of today are bumps in the road. They benefit by shutting off their senses one by one in the same manner of my proven sleep technique shared in Virgo. Libras need a comforter that is beautiful to them in some way. It has to take their breath away every time they see it or they will get a new one, something they do more than any other sign.

SCORPIO

Scorpios need sexual activity to help them fall asleep. If that is not practical, then they should know that the benefits of their descent into the arms of Morpheus will lead them to having their usual night of intense and, you guessed it, sexual dreams. They need a comforter that is sexy in some way—that has a look and feel to it that is conducive to their intense experience of life.

SAGITTARIUS

Sagittarians can fall asleep by either using sleep techniques used by other cultures—and they all have them—or by visualizing people doing so all around the world. They should research the way various cultures sleep, how they arrange sleep areas, what, if anything, they use for pillows, and what they think happens to a person's soul when sleep overcomes them. A Sagittarius would enjoy a quilt that reminds them of a culture other than their own with which they feel an affinity, either an ethnic print or a design that is emblematic of a particular culture.

CAPRICORN

Capricorns will usually fall asleep when they know it is time to fall asleep and they will do it regularly. If their timing cycle is disturbed, they might have trouble falling asleep. They have a tendency to be quite serious and to see the stark reality that almost all the other signs prefer to push away in favor of the illusion that life is not as difficult and short as it really is. Their tendency to mull things over and possibly feel a bit depressed, especially when they are tired, suggests that they would benefit from a comforter that was cheery and bright, maybe even a bit reminiscent of a child's comforter in some way, though their respect for tradition and their desire to be respected might incline them to instead use a comforter that is traditional and of high quality with a respected brand name.

AQUARIUS

Aquarians approach sleep the way most people approach death and so they usually don't go to sleep at regular hours when regular people go to regular sleep. They may stay up too late and rarely go to bed early, unless they are not feeling well. What helps them go to sleep is to forget that they have to go to sleep—they hate being told what to do—and to let themselves be so tired that they have to go to sleep or else start becoming inefficient in their thought processes. They would certainly do well with a crazy quilt, and the crazier the better, but any comforter that is either of the past or the future would be okay with them. The truth is that they don't really care about such things because sleep is not one of their favorite things.

PISCES

Pisceans are kind of dreamy all the time, so going to sleep is usually not a problem for them unless someone around them or that they are in psychic communication with, like a sibling or a parent, is in distress. If that is the case, then they have to contact them and talk it out before sleep will be possible. They can be so sensitive that even if there's someone in a neighboring apartment who is upset, they'll feel it, so they need to do some psychic armoring exercises as part of their daily ritual. Pisces needs a comforter that is a dream in and of itself. It has to be a work of art in some way and evoke a feeling of peace, love, and tranquility.

Final Thoughts

The stars, the planets, and crystals are formed by heat and pressure—so are we all!

Life is relentless, which is why you have to be equally relentless in your dedication to make a conscious effort daily to attain the maximum level of wellness you are capable of attaining. Wellness happens when you see and treat your body, mind, and spirit like the precious best friends they are, listening to them, pampering as best you can, and doing everything in your power to enjoy a life shared in inseparable intimacy.

When it comes to wellness, if you can find pleasure in your journey, then you are halfway to your goal. One sign that you are creating wellness is the quality of the people you are attracting to yourself. If you are on that path, you are much more likely to be the kind of person who can attract to you the kind of friends and partners that you enjoy and who can add to your level of "living wellness."

Wellness may even be catching! We will always treasure the day our family doctor told us, prior to our physicals, that he strongly believed that his tests would continue to show us healthy—because his office staff always looked forward to our visits and remarked to him that our interactions with them made them feel calmer and happier. Now that is good medicine!

Wellness is so powerful, it can affect even people you have never met. We have a dear friend who, as of this writing, is fighting for her life against a very difficult illness in a most noble and inspiring way. We have had close family members who also showed us strength and resilience in the face of painful and threatening health challenges. Having such an illness, or being with someone who has, reinforces the awareness that life is so precious and fragile.

Visiting our friend at her apartment in New York City afforded us the opportunity to get to know a very nice man who works in the parking garage in the basement of her high rise. When we told him who we were there to see, he sighed deeply and told us that he had never met our friend but wanted to, because the people coming to see her were uniformly kind to him and spoke so positively of her, he knew she must be a very special person.

When we related this story to our friend she was deeply moved, and it was evident that the experience was energizing to her, because she made plans to make the difficult journey downstairs to meet him.

We get chills thinking about this beautiful exchange of love, vitamin "L," and it may be that love, the ultimate spiritual power tool, is the key to unlocking the inner healer and the well of wellness within each of us. If you don't have a person or a pet to love, then love yourself and see what happens. We think you'll be pleasantly surprised.

When you use your creative potential to do your best with what you have to make things the way you would like them to be, you are no longer a victim. You are, instead, living your life to the fullest.

Remind yourself daily to give thanks and show your gratitude for all that you have. Send healing energy and whatever clarity you can share out into the world. Keep your sense of humor and your sense of proportion as you seek to become yourself fully. Put each person you meet at the center of your world and theirs. Many blessings to you, and may you seek and find contentment in all circumstances.

About the Authors

MONTE FARBER AND AMY ZERNER

Internationally known self-help author Monte Farber's inspiring guidance and empathic insights impact everyone he encounters. Amy Zerner's exquisite, one-of-a-kind spiritual couture clothing creations and collaged fabric paintings exude her profound intuition and deep connection with archetypal stories and healing energies.

Amy is an Aries and Monte is an Aquarius. For more than forty years they've combined their deep love for each other with the work of inner exploration and self-discovery to build The Enchanted World of Amy Zerner & Monte Farber: astrology books, tarot card decks, and oracles that have helped millions answer questions, be more mindful, find deeper meaning, and follow their own spiritual paths.

Together they've made their love for each other a work of art and their art the work of their lives. Their bestselling titles include *Karma Cards: A Guide to Your Future Through Astrology*, *Sun Sign Secrets*, *Signs & Seasons: An Astrology Cookbook*, *The Soulmate Path*, *The Psychic Circle*, *The Chakra Meditation Kit*, *The Enchanted Tarot*, *The Enchanted Spellboard*, *Little Reminders: The Law of Attraction*, *Instant Tarot*, *The Truth Fairy*, *Tarot Secrets*, and *Quantum Affirmations*.

Their websites are www.AmyZerner.com, www.MonteFarber.com, and www.TheEnchantedWorld.com.

Index